FROM STUCK
TO
Unstuck

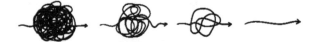

**BREAK FREE FROM THE OCD & ANXIETY
LOOP USING THE TRIPLE-A RESPONSE®
AND TAKE BACK CONTROL OF YOUR LIFE**

First paperback edition October 2023

Book design by Kirk Sta. Ana

ISBN 979-8-9892181-0-3 (eBook)
ISBN 979-8-9892181-1-0 (paperback)

www.restoredminds.com

Before you get started...

I want to give you access to our From Stuck to Unstuck Toolkit, which will enhance your understanding and application of everything you will learn in this book. Plus, as a special bonus, we're including an audiobook version of the book to make it even more accessible and convenient for you.

This exclusive toolkit equips you with a powerful set of resources to help you gain the clarity you need to move towards your recovery with complete confidence.

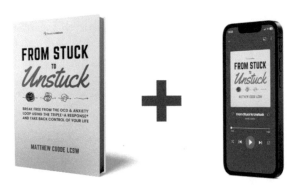

What's Inside the Toolkit?

- FREE Audiobook Version
- 10 Powerful Training Videos
- Engaging Exercises
- OCD & Anxiety Assessments
- Additional Bonus Resources

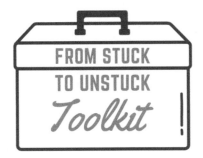

And the best thing is, it's FREE! So <u>visit the link below</u> to gain access to the toolkit and don't miss out on this exclusive opportunity.

restoredminds.com/toolkit

Contents

Dedication

This book is dedicated to anyone who currently struggles or has struggled with the challenges of being stuck in the OCD & anxiety loop. I know all too well the pain and anguish of being stuck in that loop and the impact it can have on your life. That said, I also know that you can break free from that loop. Yes, you read that correctly. **You can break free**. And I truly hope the information in this book will help you start taking the correct steps on your journey toward finding freedom.

Disclaimer

The content in this book is meant to offer information and proven strategies to assist the purchaser in coping with common symptomology associated with OCD and anxiety-related disorders. The author of this book has applied the methods described within to help himself and many of his clients achieve positive results.

Reading this book does not guarantee that the reader's results will emulate the author's results or other clients' results. The author has made all reasonable efforts to provide current and accurate information for the readers. The author does not assume any responsibility for errors, omissions, or contrary interpretations of the subject matter herein. The author further assumes no responsibility or liability and specifically disclaims any warranty, expressed or implied, for any products or services mentioned or any techniques or practices described. Additionally, any perceived slight of specific people or organizations is unintentional.

The material in this book may include information, opinions, methods, or services used by third parties. Third-Party materials are comprised of the opinions expressed by their owners. As such, the author of this book does not assume responsibility or liability for any third-party material or opinions.

No part of this publication shall be reproduced, transmitted, or resold in whole, in part, or in any form without the author's prior written consent. All trademarks and registered trademarks appearing in the book, including, the Triple-A Response®, are the author's property.

Due to the serious nature of the subject of mental health, this book is not intended as a substitute for the medical advice of physicians. The reader should regularly consult a physician and trained mental health practitioners in matters relating to their health, particularly concerning any symptoms that may require diagnosis or medical attention. The self-help resources in this book and the corresponding Restored Minds website are not a substitute for individual therapy or professional advice.

The self-help content offered in this book is solely the author's opinion. It should not be considered a form of therapy, advice, direction, diagnosis, or treatment of any kind: medical, spiritual, mental, or other. If expert advice or counseling is needed, the services of a competent professional should be sought by the reader. The reader of this self-help publication assumes full responsibility for the use of these materials and information.

Lastly, the persons, quotes, and case examples in this book are based on people the author has spoken to and interacted with on a personal or professional basis. Pseudonyms are used for all the case examples in this book to protect privacy. Disguised physical descriptions have also been used to protect each individual's identity.

All scientific research and third-party information are fully referenced for each chapter in the endnotes. Any readers, listeners, or consumers of this book are welcome to contact me for further information. You may reach me through my website: **www.restoredminds.com.** I welcome any comments, questions, or concerns.

Acknowledgments

The creation of this book would not have been possible without the support of many people along my journey. I want to express my sincere and deepest gratitude to everyone who has helped—in any capacity—along the way. You are part of the team that made this all possible.

Introduction

Welcome to the book, From Stuck to Unstuck. I want to start by congratulating you on taking a major step toward getting your life back from OCD and anxiety. I'm sure you are filled with many feelings right now, like fear, excitement, self-doubt, and maybe even some cautious optimism. And all of that is totally normal and completely OK.

As you'll soon discover, I have the intention of communicating with you in a very honest and transparent, maybe even blunt, fashion through the pages of this book. I believe it is the best way that I can help people who are stuck in the OCD & anxiety loop. Time is of the essence in this situation, which is why I have done my best to remove all the fluff and get straight to the point to help get you results. So let me begin by telling you the reasons this book exists in the first place:

Reason #1

To reduce your risks while learning how to implement a new method that I believe will help you. By design, this book won't take long to read, and it'll only set you back the price of a cup of coffee! I want you to experience as little risk as possible with a potential massive reward.

Reason #2

To provide you with a great deal of value upfront so you can start getting results quickly. This will enable you to see the benefits of this method right from the offset.

Reason #3

By accomplishing reasons 1 and 2, I hope that if there comes the point where you decide to invest in yourself and work with someone to help you implement what you have learned on a deeper level, you will choose to work with me and my team at Restored Minds, so we can help you achieve the best results possible.

Now, to accomplish all of that, I've structured this book as follows:

- In the first section, I want you to get a complete picture of the OCD & anxiety loop. We will discuss the nervous system and the four main components of the loop, then explore how the loop works. We will also discuss how and why you get stuck in the loop and what that experience is like. That way, using this foundation, I can give you specific guidance and advice through this book to help you break out of the loop.

- In the second section, I will discuss the most common challenges people face with the OCD & anxiety loop and make a clear case for using The Triple-A Response® as your primary tool to break the loop. Through this section, I hope it will become evident to you why the Triple-A Response® is the solution you need to implement for most of your OCD and anxiety struggles.

- In the third section, we will explore how to apply the Triple-A Response® to your life. I will break down the three steps of the process while providing examples of how to use them and various analogies to develop your understanding of how to implement each step.

The goal of this book is plain and simple. I want anyone currently stuck in the OCD & anxiety loop to understand and apply the Triple-A Response® consistently in their life by the end of the book.

It might sound like a lot, but really, I can sum up the entire book in the following three points:

1. How you understand any problem in life will determine what you do, and what you do will produce specific results. Therefore, if you don't currently have the desired results, you should start by ensuring you understand the problem correctly.

2. The OCD & anxiety loop is not a thought or feeling problem; it is a loop problem. This loop is fueled by engaging in safety behaviors.

3. Your primary objective for recovery is to break the loop. The best (and only) way to do this is by eliminating all your safety behaviors—mental and physical. And the best way I know how to do that is to move to a solution-focused approach called the Triple-A Response®.

I created this book to empower you and teach you that you do not have to be condemned to a life stuck in the OCD & anxiety loop. I designed this book to voice that it is possible to break free and live a life full of purpose and excitement, despite what anyone else may have told you up to this point.

My role in our time together has nothing to do with acting as your therapist. Rather, my role is to teach you how to become your own healer. Simply put, my part to play is to provide you with the information, suggestions, and guidance covered in this book. Your role is to put it into action. You are the hero in this story. I am simply your guide. I am your guide because I have walked the path before you. And I hope that one day after you get to where you want to go, you will turn around and be the guide for someone else.

The method you are about to learn in this book has radically transformed my life for the better and helped many other people. I sincerely hope that you can make the connection for yourself as well.

And while this book is technically about the OCD & anxiety loop, from a higher perspective it is really a book about developing better mental health so you can live a better life—a life that brings you joy, love, excitement, opportunities, and peace.

I wholeheartedly believe that recovery and restoration are possible for everyone, and if you are reading this book, I especially believe that for you. And I want you to know that as we embark on this journey together you are a part of a story that is bigger than just you and your recovery. You are embarking on a journey that will be part of the healing of others as well.

The reality is, the healing of the whole must begin with the healing of the individual. As we heal as individuals, we become the spark and inspiration for healing in our personal relationships. And through healing our personal relationships, we can go forward to heal as families and communities. And the healing of communities will ultimately enable us to heal together as a society and world.

This is exactly why true restoration begins within and ultimately starts with you and your mind—a restored mind is truly the beginning of a restored world.

Through this book, it is a great privilege to share what I know with you. I hope it inspires and informs you to grow and improve in every way possible so you can go forth and improve the lives of others.

If you read this book and decide that you would like help implementing its strategies, please complete a free application on the link below, and my team and I will reach out and connect with you.

http://www.restoredminds.com/tbc

We're here to help.

To your success,

Matt Codde LCSW

CHAPTER ONE
Living with OCD and Anxiety

"One thing you can't hide—is when you're crippled inside."

John Lennon

Living with OCD and anxiety was one of the most debilitating experiences of my life. It was as close to a living hell as I could imagine. One of the main reasons I think OCD and anxiety is so tough is that it is always with you. It's an ongoing battle that never seems to end, a constant bombardment of intrusive thoughts and extreme surges of stress that continually hit you.

Now, most people experience random intrusive thoughts and anxious feelings from time to time. So what makes the OCD and anxiety experience different? The answer is that with OCD and anxiety, you get caught in a loop, and in that loop, intrusive thoughts and anxious feelings are constantly happening. There's no let-up.

Most people I work with agree that it's not the random thoughts or feelings that make OCD and anxiety all-consuming. It's the compounding effect of fighting with your thoughts and feelings every single hour, of every day, with no escape. This slowly wears you down at a core level. At least, this is how it was for me.

Why I Wrote This Book

There is one main message I want to bring to you in this book, one thing I want you to remember above all: While battling OCD and anxiety can be incredibly debilitating (after all, it was the most challenging thing I've ever experienced), it **doesn't have to be a life sentence**. You can break free! You can recover! No matter what your fears are or how long you've been living with them, **you can recover!**

How?

Well, It all comes down to perspective and strategy. You must develop a new understanding of the issue at hand, equip yourself with an effective action plan, and execute that plan. This is the key to overcoming your OCD and anxiety. Think of your recovery as a skill you are going to learn, a skill you just haven't learned yet!

Recovery starts with shifting your perspective. It begins by changing the way you view the problem you are struggling with. The reason for this is simple: Your understanding of the problem directly influences the actions you take to resolve it. These actions then determine the results you achieve. How can you expect to recover if the steps you're taking aren't headed in the right direction?

Therefore, a proper understanding of the issue will direct you toward the correct actions to take, which will, in turn, produce better results in your life. And while that may sound simple, it's not easy. That's exactly why I wrote this book.

I, too, have experienced overwhelming intrusive thoughts that seemed totally insurmountable. And without the help of a new perspective, a fool-proof strategy, and the support of a few good people, I'd still be there now. At this point, I'd like to share my story with you, not to complain or dwell on the past, but purely to demonstrate that I've been where you are now. I've been down the rabbit hole. I've been lost in the chaos. I've spent more time stuck in the vicious loop of intrusive thoughts than I care (or want!) to count.

This book is personal. It draws from first-hand experience and practical application from someone who's walked this path personally. I'm invested in changing the lives of people with OCD and anxiety. So, here's my story.

My Story

I was eighteen years old, just out of high school, and headed to community college. My sense of purpose and direction was nonexistent; I had no idea what I was going to do with my life. I was just going through the motions. That's when I was completely upended by OCD and anxiety.

One day in my first semester while sitting in class, seemingly out of nowhere, I began to have a bombardment of what-if thoughts flood my mind. At this point, I didn't really know what was going on. I just knew that my mind was being invaded by extremely disturbing intrusive thoughts. Thoughts I had never had before. In fact, they were so alarming that they set off a rush of physiological sensations: My heart was pounding out of my chest, I was sweating and shaking, and I felt a massive spike of adrenaline pulsing through my veins. I didn't understand what was happening. All I knew was that I was terrified and needed to get out of the classroom ASAP.

Over the next few days, the intrusive thoughts worsened. I tried to block them out and only think about good things. I attempted to fight them off in any way I could, but everything I did just seemed to increase their severity.

Intrusive thoughts can take on any form, but they usually surface as what-if thinking. These what-if thoughts are where OCD and anxiety live and breathe.

- What if I get a disease?
- What if God sends me to hell?
- What if I lose my salvation?
- What if I hurt a loved one?
- What if I do something sexually inappropriate?
- What if I snap and do something crazy?
- What if my family member dies?
- What if I mess up at work and get fired?
- What if I'm not with the right person?
- What if I become schizophrenic?
- What if my plane crashes?
- What if I lose all of my money?

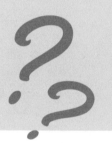

You get the idea.

My intrusive thoughts locked onto just about anything you could imagine. My mind was a breeding ground for what-if ideas. One of the thoughts that I really began spinning about was, "What if I get possessed by a demon?" This idea completely freaked me out.

Now, I had no clue about OCD and anxiety at the time. I took the content of these thoughts I was experiencing at face value and concluded that whatever my mind was saying was a real problem I needed to address. So as I operated from that level of consciousness, my focus was to make sure I wasn't going to get possessed.

Before this period of my life, I had gone to church on and off and practiced my faith, maybe haphazardly at best. But now, I shifted into full-on religious mode—all with the intention of preventing potential demonic possession. I started reading the Bible incessantly, and I wouldn't stop until I had read through a section without making any mistakes. I attended church three, sometimes four times a week because I was confident that I couldn't get possessed at church. I carried a Bible around with me almost everywhere I went. I only listened to Christian music or church sermons when I drove, and I constantly prayed throughout the day.

Now I want to be clear about something here. I am still a man of faith to this day, and I believe in God more than ever. And there is nothing wrong with any of these practices in the correct context. But the fact is **I wasn't doing these practices as an expression of faith**. I was performing these rituals for the sole purpose of feeling safe.

The problem with that was every time I engaged in these safety behaviors, I'd feel better (or safe) momentarily. There was a short period of relief. It would feel as if a huge pressure valve released all the feelings of danger in my body. Then another thought would pop up, and my anxiety would spike, and I'd perform my rituals again. And again . . . And again . . .

I also want to be clear about something else: These safety behaviors worked! If they had not worked, I wouldn't have kept doing them. Safety behaviors provided excellent temporary relief and made me feel safe, but the problem was I wasn't actually in danger. My mind was just producing an intrusive thought about an unwanted futuristic scenario. But by engaging in these safety behaviors, I was indirectly teaching my brain it was helping me stay safe, which caused an endless loop to form. More of this in the chapters to come.

In short, the more I engaged in my safety behaviors, the more frequently my brain produced the intrusive thoughts, which produced more anxiety, which led to more safety behaviors.

It got to the point where I was lost inside my head from the moment I woke up all the way until I went to sleep. As soon as I woke up, these what-if thoughts took hold of my mind. So, I'd start doing my safety behaviors to eliminate them and calm my anxiety.

The more energy I put into this loop, the more intense my intrusive thoughts became. They also began manifesting in other topics like harm, sex, relationships, driving, and existential ideas. As is the case with most people experiencing OCD and anxiety, this way of life eventually took its toll. I developed additional health problems: migraines, chest pains, and severe fatigue. I had trouble sleeping, struggled with digestive issues, and lost my sex drive, along with a whole bunch of other physical problems, all because I was in a constant state of stress.

As time went on, my life got smaller and smaller because my whole day was occupied by trying to fight with my mind. It led to the neglect and, ultimately, end of several friendships. I started getting in trouble at work. I couldn't focus in school. I isolated myself because I didn't want to be around anyone.

Eventually, I entered into a deep state of depression. I was just so tired of fighting with my mind. Every morning I told myself, "Just get through the day." It was my only goal, just to make it through the day. But after a while of just "getting through the day," I didn't want to get up and do that anymore. I didn't want to keep living like this. I wanted to have friends. I wanted to have fun. I wanted to smile again. I wanted to look forward to the day like I used to.

At this point in my journey, I had never really told anyone about what I was experiencing. I felt ashamed because I knew other people weren't living like this. I knew most people weren't consumed by worry all the time and that they definitely didn't spend all their time trying to do all these behaviors to feel safe. But I felt like I didn't have a choice—like the control of my eternal salvation was on the line.

That's another very challenging aspect of OCD and anxiety. The fight is so constant, but at the same time, it is utterly invisible to everyone else. It's like you're carrying this invisible weight around with you wherever you go. But if you do this long enough, something eventually has to give. For me, it was one night in the depths of chaos. I was crying on the floor in my room, and I finally broke and decided to get help. I wasn't sure if I was going crazy or whether I would get admitted to some locked facility. All I knew was that I couldn't keep doing what I was doing.

Over the next several months, I met with numerous therapists, counselors, and faith leaders. The general advice I received was something along the lines of . . .

"Stop worrying about it."
"You need to let this go."
"There's no point worrying about this."
"You're totally fine; this isn't real."

While these professionals were well-intentioned in their advice, their guidance didn't help me. They would offer me reassurance, which made me feel better, but only temporarily. In hindsight, most of the therapy I attended just became a new safety behavior. An expensive one too! I eventually stopped going altogether because, deep down, I just knew that none of these people truly understood what I was experiencing.

My journey's most significant turning point happened unexpectedly one day at church. I used to attend a particular church where they had people that would pray with me to stop me from getting possessed (yet another safety behavior I performed). One day, a church volunteer who was praying with me looked me straight in the eyes and said, "You know, I think you have OCD."

I was taken aback initially, and my immediate response was to correct her, so I said something like, "No, sorry, I don't wash my hands, and I don't care about germs. I don't have OCD." That just reflected how limited my understanding of OCD and anxiety was at that time. But she insisted, "Hey, I really think you should take a look and talk to someone who understands OCD and anxiety. They might be able to help you."

After that meeting, I never saw her again, but this woman literally changed the course of my life and probably saved me altogether, all with one simple sentence, offered from a place of sincere conviction and compassion. So to the woman who spoke to me that day, if by some chance you are reading this and remember talking to me, I want to say with the deepest sincerity, thank you.

Conquering OCD and Anxiety

That one day changed the trajectory of my recovery and, ultimately, my entire life. My problem wasn't due to a lack of effort, but a misunderstanding of the problem. This shift of perspective, from "this is a possession problem" to "this is an OCD and anxiety problem" set me on the course of appropriate action. As I said right at the beginning of this chapter, your understanding of the problem determines the steps you take to resolve it. And your actions determine your results.

Once I understood this, I began to recognize that my behaviors reinforced my fears. Whenever I attempted to eliminate or fight off my intrusive thoughts, avoid something that triggered me, or seek reassurance, I fed into the vicious loop.

A visible change in my life came when I shifted my focus to stopping the behaviors, not my thoughts and feelings. This was the key to my recovery. The shift allowed me to take back control over my life.

The last thing I want to leave you with is this: Today, at thirty-five years of age, I live a life I never thought possible when I was stuck in that loop. I have a beautiful wife, Jessica, and we have an amazing daughter, Jacqueline. They are my world. I have better and more authentic friendships than I've ever had in my life. I get to spend great quality time with my parents and my brother. I've had the opportunity to travel the world. I started my company, Restored Minds, where I get the chance to work with people struggling with OCD and anxiety and help them with their recovery.

And most importantly, I love being alive. I am excited to wake up. I feel so blessed and grateful to experience all that life has to offer.

I would never have believed you if you had told me, when I was in the depths of OCD and anxiety, that my life was going to look like this. When I was stuck, I felt hopeless—life felt like a constant battle that I just had to survive. Life felt heavy, like something that had to be endured. Of course, I still have challenges and struggles; those are part of life. But overall, I truly love being alive, and I genuinely look forward to my future. This still amazes me to this day, because there was a time when I never thought that would be possible.

And here's the important thing I want you to understand: **the same is possible for you**. If you feel like there's no hope, if you feel weighed down by your OCD and anxiety, if you feel like you're in quicksand with nothing to grab onto, I get it. I've been there. Please know that hope is always there, even if you can't see it, even if you've been suffering from these intrusive thoughts and anxious feelings for years or decades. You *can* break out. Recovering from OCD and anxiety is about developing a new understanding of the problem and equipping yourself with a strategy to break yourself out of the loop.

So that's what I intend to give you with this book. I want you to leave with a new understanding of what you are experiencing and a new way to approach it. That is why I'm going to teach you the Triple-A Response®, a solution-focused strategy that WILL, help you break free from OCD and anxiety. But before we do that, the first step to recovery is correctly understanding the problem, the OCD & anxiety loop. This is what I'll cover next, so meet me over in the next chapter.

CHAPTER TWO

The OCD & Anxiety Loop

"A problem well stated is a problem half solved."

Charles Franklin Kettering

When you're stuck in the OCD & anxiety loop, you rarely see the problem as being trapped in the loop. Instead, you perceive the problem as a specific thought or situation you're afraid of. This could be germs, poor health, relationships, panic attacks, social gatherings, fear of causing harm, fear of acting sexually inappropriately, fear of going to hell, etc. The list could go on and on. But as I said in chapter one, how you perceive the problem determines the actions you take to resolve it. Your actions will then dictate your results. If you see the problem as a fearful object/person/situation, you will attempt to solve that, not the actual root cause. This results in the OCD & anxiety loop forming.

So what's the real problem you are experiencing?

When we face OCD, anxiety, and other forms of psychological stress, the problem is the fear itself, not the actual thing you're afraid of. In the words of Franklin D. Roosevelt in his 1933 First Inaugural Address, "The only thing we have to fear is fear itself." There is a wealth of wisdom to unpack from this simple sentence.

If you are reading this book, I'm sure you're aware that living in fear stops you dead in your tracks, just like a deer in headlights. Fear wears you down physically, mentally, emotionally, and spiritually. It makes you operate from the lowest, most primal state of your consciousness. As we will discuss in the next chapter, fear can be very helpful if you're in an actual dangerous situation because, at that moment, you need quick, fast-paced decisions to keep yourself alive. The primal brain is excellent at this (Bessel van der Kolk, 2014). But if you're not in an actual dangerous situation, this system leads to poor decision-making that doesn't align with your long-term desires.

I wholeheartedly believe that OCD, anxiety, and other forms of psychological stress are the source of a lot of the (perceived) problems we face in today's society. And the primary reason for this: We never see fear as the issue. We are entirely blind to it. We live our lives bouncing from one topic of fear to the next, lost in our minds, living in a constant state of psychological stress. The longer this goes unnoticed, the larger the grip fear has on our lives. It grows and grows to the point where it controls every aspect of our existence. So I believe President Roosevelt was right; living in fear is the only thing we should really be afraid of. Because when we are living in fear, we are usually unaware of it.

The OCD & Anxiety Loop

The OCD & anxiety loop has four key components:

These four elements, intrusive thoughts, uncomfortable feelings, safety behaviors, and temporary relief when activated together, create a loop, as you can see in the image. When broken down, here's what the loop looks like: An intrusive thought occurs, which stirs up an uncomfortable feeling in your body. This

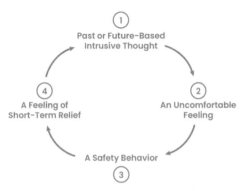

1. Past or Future-Based Intrusive Thought

2. An Uncomfortable Feeling

3. A Safety Behavior

4. A Feeling of Short-Term Relief

uncomfortable feeling causes you to engage in a safety behavior, something you do (mentally or physically) to avoid, check, control, or reassure yourself in order to neutralize the uncomfortable feeling or feared situation/object/person. This makes the uncomfortable feeling go away, but only temporarily. Shortly after the period of relief, an intrusive thought pops up again and the cycle repeats.

This may be the same intrusive thought as before, or a different one entirely. The new intrusive thought triggers more uncomfortable feelings, which lead to you performing another safety behavior. And the wheel keeps spinning.

This is what it's like for a person caught in the loop. There's an endless cycle of intrusive fearful thoughts that cause stress and anxiety, followed by the temporary relief offered by safety behaviors. If this crippling cycle isn't dealt with properly, it can take over your entire life.

But what drives the loop? The simple answer is fear. Fear is the driving force of the loop. To really understand this, we need an example. A bread-and-butter case study depicting the OCD & anxiety loop is a fear of contamination or contracting an illness.

Usually, in this instance, the first thing to happen is the individual experiencing an "external trigger." This is perceived as something in the world outside of one's body. Let's say, in this case, that an individual touches a doorknob. Then, after touching the doorknob, their mind begins to produce a few what-if scenarios, such as, "What if that doorknob has germs on it?" This is an example of an *internal trigger* in response to the *external trigger*.

KEY POINTS

In this scenario, you have a person that is not in any present danger, and their mind is creating a futuristic unwanted scenario which in turn activates their nervous system.

The external trigger was the act of touching the doorknob.

The internal trigger was the thought, "What if that doorknob has a disease on it?"

But generally, you don't just get one what-if intrusive thought. Often, what-if thoughts travel in packs. So, "What if that doorknob has a disease on it?" could quickly be followed by the following:

- "What if I have a disease on my hand?"
- "What if I become infected by that disease?"
- "What if that disease is deadly?"
- "What if I die from the disease?"
- "What if I spread that disease to my family?"

You get the idea . . .

These what-if intrusive thoughts set off the individual's stress response, which is simply the nervous system telling the body they are in a challenging or threatening situation. This is commonly referred to as the *fight-or-flight response*. When this response is activated, the person begins to feel a surge of energy in the body—this is the uncomfortable feeling in the loop. As these anxious feelings surface throughout the body, the individual feels compelled to do something to solve the problem. In this case, they might feel the urge to wash their hands.

Now, once the individual washes their hands, they generally experience a huge flood of immediate relief. The nervous system will calm down, and all the stress energy in the body will seem to vanish. But through this shift in energy, the brain and nervous system learned two things: (1) the act of washing hands kept me safe, and (2) doorknobs must really be dangerous. So shortly after, the individual will encounter another external trigger (doorknob) that will set the whole process off again. This is how the loop forms.

Let's go back to the external trigger. Notice how, in this example, the only thing that happened was that the person touched a doorknob. The doorknob didn't cause the stress response to go off. If that were true, everyone who touched that doorknob would have their stress response go off. Instead, the stress response was activated due to the "what-if" thoughts in the individual's mind, coupled with the beliefs, perceptions, and conditioning associated with the thoughts.

It is very important to understand that distinction and realize that internal triggers drive the stress response more than external triggers. The reason this is important goes back to the foundational principle of this book about how you understand this problem. If you believe your external triggers are the problem, you will try to eliminate all of your external triggers out in the world, and that will lead to a very limited life.

This one idea leads many people to go through their life fearing and avoiding doorknobs.

Getting Stuck in the OCD & Anxiety Loop

Now, if you wrestle with OCD and anxiety, you likely have experienced the frequency and intensity of intrusive thoughts worsen over time. This is due to the fact that all the safety behaviors you engage in reinforce the loop associated with the specific intrusive thought. Every time you engage in a safety behavior, you communicate to your brain and nervous system that "there is a real problem here that I need to solve." And the feeling of relief after the safety behavior is performed only serves to further reinforce this. Therefore, the loop gets worse over time. This pattern of reinforcement is a perfect example of classical conditioning.

Classical Conditioning

Have you ever heard of Pavlov's dogs? Well, if not, in the 1890s, Russian physiologist Ivan Pavlov conducted studies on dogs, looking at reinforcing behaviors (McLeod, 2020). Pavlov noticed that the sight of food caused dogs to salivate, so he began ringing a bell each time he presented the dogs with food. Over time, Pavlov stopped providing food and only rang the bell. He found that the dogs salivated at the bell, even when he didn't present any food. The dogs' brains had made a connection between the bell and food, and through repetition, Pavlov was able to activate a physiological change (salivation) in the dog's body by ringing the bell. Pretty amazing when you think about it. This is called *classical conditioning*.

This is precisely how your nervous system works. We can become conditioned to fear something by repeating behaviors that reinforce the idea that it's dangerous. So as I said earlier with the example of contamination fears, by engaging in repetitive safety behaviors, the individual's nervous system and brain are learning two specific things:

1. Washing their hands kept them safe.
2. The doorknob is dangerous.

Now, was the doorknob actually dangerous?

Did washing their hands keep them safe?

Short answer—no.

Longer answer—we can never truly be certain, as certainty doesn't exist. As humans, we have to live and operate in the laws of probability, and it is highly improbable any real danger was encountered by touching the doorknob. Therefore, it is highly unlikely that the act of washing their hands increased their safety.

Now let's dig a little deeper. Was the actual problem in this scenario a disease problem or a fear of disease problem? The individual perceived it as a disease problem based on their what-if thoughts, so that's what they tried to solve: a disease problem. By going through this process repetitively, their brain began to believe that their what-if thoughts are valid and help keep them safe. Which, in turn, makes them more fearful of doorknobs. This is a misperception, resulting in the person engaging in more safety behaviors that will reinforce the OCD & anxiety loop.

And the fear of contamination is just one of many manifestations a person can experience.

Common Types of Fears

As you probably know, the OCD & anxiety loop can manifest with many different types of fears. It can also shift at times into various themes. In fact, in my experience, most people experience multiple different loops throughout their life.

Let's go through some of the most common subtypes of OCD & anxiety loops people can get caught up in. Some common fears include the following:

- Contamination
- Emotional contamination
- Specific diseases
- Real events
- False memories
- Having a panic attack
- Feeling anxiety
- Health and bodily functions
- Bodily sensations
- Social situations
- Relationships/loved ones
- Intrusive/unwanted harmful thoughts
- Intrusive/unwanted sexual thoughts
- Religious doubts or existential ideas
- Fears about God or the afterlife
- Going to specific places
- Certain numbers and/or symbols
- Losing control
- Something terrible happening
- Orderliness and perfection
- Driving or flying

Now, the second half of the loop consists of the safety behaviors a person performs to eliminate the uncomfortable feeling caused by the thoughts. There are also numerous types of safety behaviors one can engage in. Let's go through some of the common safety behaviors below.

Common Types of Safety Behaviors

Safety behaviors fall into two broad categories: physical and mental. A physical safety behavior is when you perform a physical action to avoid, cope, check, or reassure yourself, resulting in temporary relief. A mental safety behavior works in the same way but is performed internally.

Let's take a look at common examples of both.

Common Physical Safety Behaviors

- Avoiding triggering shows, movies, or songs
- Avoiding triggering places
- Avoiding triggering people
- Avoiding triggering objects
- Seeking reassurance from websites, articles, or videos
- Seeking verbal reassurance from a loved one
- Repetitive checking (locks, stove, etc.)
- Using substances (alcohol/marijuana)
- Excessive showering and washing
- Repetitive grooming or bodily hygiene routines
- Attempting to control other people's behaviors
- Setting up controlling rules
- Engaging in repetitive schedules or routines

Common Mental Safety Behaviors

- Overanalyzing
- Mental checking
- Mental rumination
- Mentally trying to solve something or "figure it out"
- Mental reassurance
- Mentally checking for thoughts/feelings
- Excessive body scanning
- Trying to distract yourself
- Thought blocking
- Thought replacement
- Thought suppression
- Silent prayer
- Mentally counting
- Repetition of specific phrases/verses

It's important to understand that all safety behaviors are actions used to alleviate the stress generated after the initial what-if thought. It makes no difference whether the safety behavior is mental or physical.

Let's be clear here. There are *many* safety behaviors, not just the ones on this list. More importantly, a lot of behaviors can turn into safety behaviors if you aren't careful. As I explained in the first chapter, even going to therapy can become a safety behavior.

Once the OCD & anxiety loop has gained momentum, safety behaviors become more and more frequent. All of a sudden, you're living in a constant state of fear, always in survival mode. And like we have discussed, living in a state of constant fear is one of the greatest tragedies in life.

Why You NEED to Break Out of the OCD & Anxiety Loop

Unfortunately, the OCD & anxiety loop rarely just goes away on its own. And when you are stuck in the loop, you gradually begin to lose things from your life. But you tend to overlook these losses because they happen slowly, over a prolonged period. You may not realize it, but when you're stuck in the loop, you're losing three key things every single day:

1. Opportunities
2. Time
3. Peace

Let's start with lost opportunities.

When I was stuck in the OCD & anxiety loop, I wasn't very aware of how often I said no to opportunities. I said no to things because I was preoccupied with my fear. I can recall quite clearly, how I would sit at home alone on Saturday nights for months and months. I would say no to opportunities because I felt like I needed to stay home and do my rituals, just to be sure. This resulted in me spending a lot of time in isolation and forgoing many amazing opportunities available to me at that time.

Ask yourself, how many opportunities have you missed out on due to performing safety behaviors? Are you neglecting relationships? Are there trips and vacations you've said no to? Job opportunities? When we're in the OCD & anxiety loop, we let fear decide the direction of our lives. Fear takes the driver's seat, and we become a passenger. And over time, we end up passing up amazing opportunities because we're so busy trying to feel safe.

That's what often makes the OCD & anxiety loop so debilitating. It actually isn't the thoughts and feelings that cause us to suffer. It's that we wholeheartedly believe that if we don't do our safety behaviors, it will lead to imminent doom. Our beliefs and perceptions about our thoughts and feelings is the real problem.

So we tell ourselves, "If I avoid this, check that, or get reassurance one more time, that will be enough, and *then* I'll live the life I want to live." But answer me this—when has that ever happened? When has the safety behavior ever been "enough." How many times have you told yourself, "Tomorrow will be the day I start living how I want to live," only to never see tomorrow come? How long will you continue to say no to life so you can keep chasing the feeling of safety? When will it be the right time to start taking back control?

That brings us to point number two: lost time. As my OCD & anxiety loop gained momentum, I became increasingly anxious about experiencing disturbing intrusive thoughts. I spent more and more time trying to control my thoughts. I started to notice that weeks, months, and then years were going by, and I was stuck in the same place I had always been. I watched my friends go off to college, enjoy relationships, get married, pursue jobs, go on adventures, and have all these incredible life experiences. They were taking advantage of all the opportunities I was passing on. That's when I realized what I was sacrificing. I wasn't just giving up opportunities; time was slipping away from me too.

Time is the most precious asset we have. We all have a start and end time on this earth, and no one knows for sure how many days they have between those two points. And like any other asset, you can choose how you invest your time. Every second you invest in your OCD & anxiety loop performing your safety behaviors is a poor investment because there is never a positive return. It always produces a loss that you can't get back. Many people (like myself) have invested years of their lives in this fear loop. Years they can never get back.

So ask yourself this question, am I ready to stop giving away my most precious asset to my fear?

The final thing the OCD & anxiety loop takes from you is your peace. It takes the smile off your face. That's the best way I can explain it—it simply drains the light, joy, and excitement out of everything you do. It's like walking around with a thousand-pound weight on your shoulders that no one can see. It literally impacts everything.

Even when you use safety behaviors to try to counteract it, it just comes back with a vengeance. The thoughts and feelings grow in their intensity. The more this happens, the less you want to go do things, like interact with people and engage in activities for fun. The longer the loop goes, the more it drains the peace out of you. There's a whole biological explanation for this that we will cover in the next chapter.

However, I'm not bringing all this up to make you feel bad or rain on your parade. On the contrary, it's to shine a light on the real problem because that's the biggest misunderstanding when it comes to OCD and anxiety. Most people are trying to solve the wrong problem, which prevents them from getting the results they want. The loop is the problem, *period*. The loop keeps you in a state of stress. And when you live in a chronic state of stress, you begin to see the world in a negative light. The world is not the problem; you are just misperceiving it that way. It's like you have a lens covering your eyes and distorting your view of the world. I call this the lens of fear, and it's what the next chapter is all about. See you there.

CHAPTER THREE
The Stress Response and the Lens of Fear

*"Nothing in life is to be feared, it is only to be understood.
Now is the time to understand more, so that we may fear less."*

Marie Curie

In this chapter, I will give you a quick overview of the biology of the stress response and the nervous system. But this is by no means a complete breakdown of the stress response. There are plenty of highly detailed resources out there if you wish to pursue this topic further. I just feel it's necessary to, at the very least, scratch the surface of the stress response because it will be foundational to your success through the rest of the book. Let's dive in!

The Nervous System

The most primal instinct we possess as humans is the instinct to stay alive. That is the number one function of the nervous system, to keep you alive and safe. Our brains and bodies are designed to survive. And, let's be honest, they're really good at it. Since the dawn of man, we have automatically responded to perceived danger, emergency, and/or threat in a very instinctual manner.

For instance, if you encountered a pack of wolves on your next walk, your brain and body would instantly activate your stress response and you would feel a surge of energy through your body to help you fight the wolves or run away from them. The most primitive part of your brain, the *primal* or *reptilian brain*, is in charge of these instinctual, automatic thinking and behavioral patterns (Satpute et al., 2015).

I find it helpful to view your nervous system like a giant communication system, constantly allowing all the different parts of your body to talk to each other to make sure you stay safe. Now, the nervous system is divided into two main branches: the *sympathetic nervous system*, which activates your body to respond to potential threats, and the *parasympathetic nervous system*, which slows and calms your body down. In fact, the parasympathetic nervous system actually divides into two different functions for the body, which we will discuss a little later.

When your nervous system is confident that you are safe, your body naturally begins returning to internal balance (or homeostasis). This in turn allows you to experience an open and present state of awareness where you are present to consciously engage in whatever you are doing.

Your Internal Stoplight

(This is primarily drawn from Dr. Stephen Porges and his work on polyvagal theory).

To keep it simple, to understand how your nervous system works, let's use the analogy of an upside-down stoplight, with green being at the top (parasympathetic), yellow in the middle (sympathetic), and red at the bottom (parasympathetic). Essentially this upside stoplight's job is to keep you safe, and it corresponds with the nervous system throughout different regions of your body.

As the nervous system receives information, it enters a certain state (Green, Yellow, Red) to help you navigate that situation. As it shifts from state to state, our experiences, perceptions, and feelings about the world will generally change, corresponding to that state. So when we are in Green (safety), we will usually have "green" thoughts, perceptions, and feelings of the environment and our surroundings. When we are in Yellow (danger/fight or flight), we will usually have "yellow" thoughts, perceptions, and feelings of the environment and our surroundings. And when we are in Red (freeze/shut down), we have "red" thoughts, perceptions, and feelings.

Let's do a quick breakdown of the common experiences in each state.

Green/Safety

When your nervous system is in Green, you will notice more energy directed into your face and be able to place your attention safely toward your environment. You will naturally engage in the present moment in a more open and peaceful state. You may feel in flow state or harmony. You may feel emotions such as joy, love, and happiness. You will feel connected socially to people in your life. This is where you will interact best with others and with situations, which makes sense because you will feel safe to do so. This state is activated by the parasympathetic nervous system and is referred to as *ventral vagal*.

Yellow/Danger/Fight or Flight

The Yellow state is activated by the sympathetic nervous system and will put you in a mobilized state, which is often referred to as your *fight-or-flight response*. You will notice more energy directed into your chest. You will enter this state when your system perceives a threat or challenge. In this state you will experience feelings like anxiety, anger, worry, and fear and generally feel compelled to fight or flee the perceived threat or challenge.

Red State: Freeze/Shut Down

The Red state is a freeze state, sometimes referred to as *dorsal vagal*, which is also generated by the parasympathetic nervous system. In this state, you will notice more energy directed in your gut area. It is essentially a last resort of your nervous system to handle a threat or challenge. In this state you will feel frozen, shutdown, or immobilized in response to a perceived overwhelming danger. It will feel difficult to engage in basic activities, and your energy state will be low. In this state, you will experience things like sadness, loneliness, hopelessness, and depression.

Now let me clarify something: None of these states are bad. They all serve a specific purpose, and we cycle between the Green, Yellow, and Red states every day. For instance, when you work out, you enter into Yellow. When you sleep, you enter into Red.

But as we learned last chapter, we condition the brain and nervous system through our behavior, and we can wind up stuck in loops that perpetuate us in a chronic state of stress.

The Stress Response

Now stress is something that we all experience in life. Stress is simply our body's response to a perceived challenge or demand. It is just our body shifting into Yellow. When your brain and nervous system detect danger, your body releases a bunch of hormones that stimulate the sympathetic nervous system. The activation of the sympathetic nervous system triggers a whole load of physiological changes in your body. Your heart rate increases, muscles tense, pupils dilate, vision sharpens, awareness intensifies, and blood is redirected into your limbs to help you run faster and fight more effectively. This is why you will feel more energy in your chest.

Now when you shift into Yellow, it also has an effect on your brain. According to Dr. Stephen Porges's polyvagal theory (Porges and Dana, 2018), activation of the sympathetic nervous system (Yellow) shuts down higher cognitive functions—logic is switched off, complex decision-making is down, and you can't see different perspectives on the situation at hand. Everything looks threatening in this state—you're more likely to misread social cues and assume anger and aggression all around you. You look at everything as a potential threat. This is great for dangerous situations, but hopefully you can see how it's an issue when you're constantly living in a state of stress.

The stress response is designed as a short-term survival mechanism. It helps you get out of the situation you perceive as dangerous, either through fighting or fleeing. Once you're away from danger, the other branch of the nervous system (parasympathetic nervous system) is activated, and you go into the Green state (Won and Kim, 2016). The parasympathetic nervous system counteracts the sympathetic nervous system, returning your body to a calm state.

> **A quick tip on how to remember the different systems, just remember *para* like a parachute—a parachute stops you from falling and puts you at rest.**

The stress response has been critical to ensuring our survival. Its entire purpose is to protect our lives, and it has done so for thousands of years. When humans roamed the plains, enduring the elements and fighting off predators daily, the stress response was highly successful at ensuring our survival as a species.

But here's the thing: Humans have gotten very good at surviving—so good, in fact, that we now spend most of our time at the top of the food chain. So let's give a big shout-out and thank-you to our ancestors for that one. We're rarely hunted by predators now because we've built houses, towns, and cities to keep us safe. Many of us have electricity, running water, indoor plumbing, warm showers, and even air conditioning. Effectively, we've eliminated most of our day-to-day dangers, especially in more developed parts of the world. This means that our innate survival mechanism is becoming more and more unnecessary. But this system didn't just shut off and go away. Instead, that same energy has begun to evolve and shift into predicting potential threats, considering possible futuristic dangers, and then attempting to resolve them. This is where we run into a problem.

Common Types of Stress

Now, according to Dr. Robert Sapolski in his book, *Why Zebras Don't Get Ulcers*, there are three main types of stressors we experience in life:

1. **Sudden Acute Physical Danger:** An example of a sudden acute physical danger could be a lion running at you. This is a real danger that is happening right now, and your body will initiate the stress response and attempt to fight off or flee from the lion.

2. **Long-term Physical Challenges:** An example of long-term stress could be being stuck on a deserted island or being in some form of chronic pain. Your body would

produce the stress response in an attempt to help navigate the physical challenges of this experience.

3. **Psychological Stress:** An example of this could be your mind produces a what-if thought about some future or past based event like, "What if my plane crashes?" and your body initiates the stress response in an attempt to resolve the futuristic threat.

For most of us, psychological stress is the primary type of stress that we experience in our business.

This is a rather unique experience to human beings where you witness your mind's ability to come up with various potential bad futuristic scenarios and your body literally responds to them as if they are a real present danger.

The reality is, nowadays, the majority of our stress is purely psychological.

What do I mean by this?

Instead of encountering external physical dangers, our minds conjure up ideas that predict possible future dangers and then attempt to resolve the possible threats before they even happen. Moreover, many fears seem to have shifted from our individual survival to broader concepts like societal acceptance and approval. The problem is that when our mind produces potential negative scenarios, it actually activates the same exact survival system that we use to respond to real, present danger.

Now, when it comes to psychological stress, it might seem like a good thing, but here are a few factors I want you to consider:

1. You can't successfully predict the future. No one can. If somehow you can predict the future, please buy a ticket with the correct numbers on the next major lottery drawing (preferably with a jackpot of $100 million or more). Then tell me the next ones.

2. There are an endless number of possible threats that could happen to you. So, in theory, you could spend your whole life trying to predict dangerous scenarios, putting your body under high levels of stress, without ever actually encountering any real danger in your life. Ask yourself, can you look back on a time in your life when you were really stressed out about something and honestly say, "I am really glad that I spent all that time stressed about that situation"?

3. Since the threats are simply futuristic ideas in your mind, the issue with psychological stress is that you have the ability to be in an extremely high state of stress while simultaneously being perfectly safe in the present moment.

4. When the stress response is active, your body functions differently. This is fine if the stress response is only activated for a short period like it's supposed to be. But if you're in a chronic state of stress, this negatively impacts multiple bodily functions, leading to various problems in your life.

Unfortunately for us, our bodies and brains can't distinguish between an imagined psychological threat and a real, physical one. Whether you're worried about messing up that work presentation or standing in front of an angry pack of wolves, the "threat" activates the same exact stress response.

Now bringing this all back to the OCD & anxiety loop. When you're living with OCD, anxiety, and other forms of psychological stress, you're living in a chronic state of stress because the loop just keeps going and going. What's supposed to be a short-term solution quickly becomes a long-term problem. And after a while, this takes a toll on us physically, psychologically, emotionally, and spiritually.

Psychological Stress-Related Disorders

In Western society, when our body's sympathetic nervous system (Yellow) is activated and there is no present danger, we call this *anxiety*.

Most medical professionals are quick to categorize and label these experiences of psychological stress or anxiety into specific and separate "disorders." In fact, according to the Anxiety and Depression Association of America (ADAA), stress- and anxiety-related issues impact over forty million Americans. You may have even had one or several of these labels placed on you in your own life.

But for right now let's suspend all labels and judgments, and instead I invite you to think about psychological stress or anxiety as existing on a big spectrum that can vary in both symptoms and intensity within the Yellow section of your nervous system.

Because we all experience psychological stress to some degree, it's just about understanding what you are experiencing and how to shift out of it and get your nervous system out of Yellow and back to Green. That is the goal of this book.

So moving from top to bottom in the section below, think of each description as just an experience on the Yellow spectrum, as opposed to a disorder.

- **General Anxiety** is when you experience persistent and excessive worry about a number of different things. People with GAD may anticipate disaster and may be overly concerned about money, health, family, work, or other issues.

- **Social Anxiety** is when you experience intense anxiety or fear of being judged, negatively evaluated, or rejected in a social or performance situation.

- **Phobias** are when you experience seemingly excessive and unreasonable fears in the presence of, or in anticipation of, a specific object, place, or situation.

- **Obsessive Compulsive Disorder** is when you experience intrusive and unwanted thoughts, images, or urges that cause distress or anxiety and engage in compulsive behaviors that ease your distress or anxiety or suppress the thoughts.

- **Panic Attacks/Panic Disorder** is when you experience spontaneous, out-of-the-blue panic attacks and become very preoccupied with the fear of a recurring panic attack.

- **Post-Traumatic Stress Disorder:** is developed after experiencing or witnessing a perceived life-threatening event, like combat, a natural disaster, a car accident, or sexual assault.

- **Derealization or Depersonalization** is when you repeatedly have the feeling that you're observing yourself from outside your body, or you have a sense that things around you aren't real, or both.

When I was writing this book, my goal was to find a universal language that would be relatable. The reality is that the experience of psychological stress exists on a vast continuum of different experiences that often overlap. Most people don't experience one manifestation of psychological stress. So for the purpose of this book, I am using the general language of "OCD and anxiety," but just know that what I teach in this book applies to all forms of psychological stress.

While this evolutionary shift of the mind to try to predict futuristic threats may seem beneficial, the reality is that keeping the body in a constant state of stress can cause bodily harm over time. Just like if a car engine was running 24/7, eventually, you are going to experience problems. Think back to the OCD & anxiety loop we discussed in the last chapter and all of those what-if intrusive thoughts. Each what-if thought can trigger the stress response, and essentially, they can activate your survival mechanism constantly!

You may be inclined to argue that there are, in fact, many dangerous things in the world and that you have good reason to fear them because it helps to keep you alive. But as author Paulo Coelho stated in his book *The Alchemist*, "The fear of suffering is worse than the suffering itself." In other words, it'll cause you more harm stressing about a potential threat than it would to actually deal with it head-on if and when it presents itself. And in most cases, that is a big *if* because the reality is that probably 99.99 percent of the psychological threats our minds produce never even happen. Just ask yourself, how many times has your fearful mind been right?

Living in the Lens of Fear

Okay, building off of everything we have discussed so far, let's dive into the main point of this chapter. When you experience a high amount of stress, you literally see the world in a distorted way because your nervous system is in Yellow. And when the OCD & anxiety loop is in full swing, you are in a continuous state of Yellow. This means you are experiencing the world in a distorted fashion.

When I try to explain the experience to someone who has never gone through it, I often tell them it's like wearing a pair of fear goggles at all times. When you are lost in the OCD & anxiety loop, it creates an invisible lens between you and the world, distorting your perception and making you see life completely differently from people not wearing the fear goggles.

When you are in the OCD & anxiety loop, you effectively put the goggles on automatically. You become hypervigilant, considering almost everything in your environment a potential threat. Your view of your external world suddenly and drastically changes.

But there's one key difference between putting on a pair of goggles and living through the lens of fear. If it was an actual pair of goggles, you would know you were wearing them, and you could take them off whenever you wanted.

Unfortunately, the lens of fear doesn't work that way. When you're stuck in the OCD & anxiety loop, the continual state of stress you're in makes you unaware that your view is distorted. In fact, you may even question other people's perceptions if they differ from your own. Perhaps you'll also question why no one else seems to see what you see. But you need to remember that when you are in Yellow, it bypasses your rational mind, exaggerates your fears, and distorts your thinking. These fear goggles, while they might be invisible, are very real. And as I said previously, you often never realize they are there. That's the tricky part about them. But they are real, and if you aren't careful, they can become integral to how you view the world.

So what's the point of all of this?

Well, being stuck in the lens of fear poses three serious problems:

1. You can't see the lens, so you usually don't know you're in it.

2. When you see the world through the lens of fear, you see danger everywhere, and the threats look very real.

3. Unlike real goggles, you can't physically take the fear goggles off. The fear goggles are a secondary effect of being stuck in Yellow and stuck in the OCD & anxiety loop. The only way to get the fear goggles off is by breaking out of the OCD & anxiety loop.

It's very challenging to understand the concept of the lens of fear unless you've experienced it first-hand. If you're lucky enough not to have experienced it before, please understand that once you're stuck in the OCD & anxiety loop, the lens of fear will surely develop. And it will absolutely distort your entire world.

Better Call Saul

The best depiction I have ever seen of the lens of fear is in the AMC series *Better Call Saul*. The main character, Saul, has an older brother, Chuck McGill. Chuck is a well-respected, highly successful lawyer. But when we first meet Chuck, we quickly realize something's not right. On the surface, he looks healthy. But we come to learn that he is entirely housebound. He's cut off all electricity to his suburban home, cooks on a campfire stove in his living room, and occasionally wraps himself in a tinfoil blanket. (From a clinical perspective, these are usually bad signs.) He has food delivered that is kept in a cooler on ice, lives by candlelight and gas lantern, no longer works at his firm, and only interacts with a few trusted individuals. Chuck does all this because he believes he has developed a rare allergy to electricity. As a result, he is consumed by the fear of electricity exposure.

In the series, there is an incredible scene that, I feel, really captures what it's like to be in the lens of fear. Chuck is forced to run outside to grab a newspaper. When he steps outside, you see his extreme hyperawareness of the electricity around him. Chuck notices every telephone wire, phone, and streetlight. He runs as fast as he can, wrapped in his tinfoil blanket. He grabs the newspaper and runs back into his house, all while his perplexed neighbor watches from her window.

You see, Chuck's mind and nervous system were communicating that there was a real threat to his life. His brain thought he was putting himself in a life-threatening situation by exposing himself to electricity. But there wasn't any real threat; it was a perceived threat, which created real stress in his body. This is a perfect example of psychological stress. Chuck reinforces this idea by avoiding the outside world and engaging in his other safety behaviors. In this way, he feeds into his OCD & anxiety loop and continues to live through the lens of fear.

Remember in the previous chapter we spoke about classical conditioning? In this example, Chuck reinforced the idea that the outside world was dangerous by keeping himself inside his home. What *Better Call Saul* never explains is how all this started. But I'd bet if his character is like most people in the loop, it probably all began with a single what-if intrusive thought. And through the repeated safety behaviors, the loop began to spin, the lens started to form, and this little what-if intrusive thought led to the life-altering situation we see Chuck trapped in.

SPOILER ALERT

Eventually, it's proven to the audience that Chuck doesn't actually have an allergy to electricity; it was all in his mind. He even begins to use some of the tools we will talk about in this book and completely turns his life around for a while. Unfortunately, these changes don't last for Chuck, and the ending isn't a happy one. That's what separates this show from real life—it doesn't matter that Chuck didn't succeed, because he's not real; he's just a character. You are real, and you do matter. Your story will be much different than his because you will have the right tools to be successful.

Final Thoughts

I know we bounced around a bit in this chapter, but the main point is vital to your success, so I'll state it as clearly as I can here. When you are stuck in the OCD & anxiety loop, your nervous system enters into Yellow, and a lens of fear forms over your life that radically distorts your perception of the world. You can't see this lens, but I assure you it is there. When you're in the lens of fear, you aren't seeing your real problem correctly—just like Chuck didn't really have an electricity problem and I didn't really have a demonic possession problem. We both got stuck in the OCD & anxiety loop. As a result, the lens of fear developed and distorted our views of the world. Which led to both of us living a very limited life. And in the same way, you don't have the problem your mind is telling you have. You have an OCD & anxiety loop problem.

Here's the reality: When it comes to OCD and anxiety, the odds of your fear actually happening are probably slim to none, and even if it were to occur, the suffering caused by the feared event would be far less than the continual stress of attempting to prevent it from happening. The real suffering comes from being stuck in the loop itself. When you're caught in the lens, the object/person/situation you fear looks like the problem. But the *real* problem is living in fear. As I explained in the last chapter, living in fear leads to losing opportunities, time, and peace. And when you think about it, those are some of the most important things we have in this life.

The loop is what keeps your nervous system in Yellow and strengthens the lens of fear over your life. The lens of fear distracts you from seeing the loop as the problem, and that is how you remain stuck. But once you break the loop, your nervous system shifts back into Green, and the lens begins to lift. Once that happens, you begin to see the world clearly again. How do you break the loop? By eliminating all of your safety behaviors. And to do that, you have to first make a few important shifts. Don't worry, I'll guide you through this in chapter four. See you there.

CHAPTER FOUR

Three Critical Shifts

"Everyone thinks of changing the world, but no one thinks of changing himself."

Leo Tolstoy

One of my all-time favorite movies is *Moneyball*, and I think the story of *Moneyball* has a weird parallel with OCD and anxiety recovery. Let me explain for those of you who haven't seen the movie. There's one particular scene that I feel really highlights how most people veer off course when it comes to understanding OCD and anxiety. In this specific scene, the character Peter Brand (played by Jonah Hill) is talking to the Oakland Athletics general manager Billy Beane (played by Brad Pitt) in an underground parking lot. They're having this private conversation out of the office because they don't want to be overheard. During the conversation, Peter Brand says the following:

There is an epidemic failure within the game to understand what is really happening. And this leads people who run Major League Baseball teams to misjudge their players and mismanage their teams.

He goes into more detail, explaining that people who run professional baseball teams focus on the wrong things and analyze the wrong data points. And as a result, they make a series of bad decisions that negatively impact their teams and ultimately lead to unsuccessful results for the organizations.

This is how I feel about many practitioners (i.e., coaches, therapists, doctors, psychologists, and psychiatrists) who try to help people struggling with OCD and anxiety. Yes, I know this is a big controversial statement that I'm making, and I'm not saying this lightly either. You know from chapter 1 that I paid many different therapists (not to mention several other medical professionals) before a church volunteer told me I might have OCD!

Not once did any of the licensed professionals or doctors I visited suggest I was dealing with OCD and anxiety, let alone offer or direct me to an effective solution. All of them tried to talk through the content of my fear. I acknowledge that they were well-intended in their efforts to help me and offered me the best tools they had in their toolkit, but each one of them was directing me to incorrect interventions.

Now, practitioners offering incorrect guidance to problems isn't a new thing. This has gone on since the dawn of man. To prove this point, we could draw on some extreme examples, like the ancient civilizations conducting human sacrifices to convince the gods to make it rain. While we can't be certain, I have a distinct feeling that the people who were sacrificed didn't think this was the best solution for rain. Alternatively, we can draw on much more recent examples. Less than one hundred years ago, there were common mental health interventions like lobotomies and electro-shock treatment. In the late 1800s, opium and cocaine were thought to be medicine. Even Sigmund Freud, one of the pioneers of psychology, was very outspoken about his love for cocaine and all its potential "benefits." And we won't even go into things like the Tuskegee study. You can google it if you want to (but beware, it might upset you).

The point is, when you are seeking help for something, you can't just assume that the guidance you receive from someone is correct, no matter what credentials they have next to their name. Before you follow anyone's advice, and most of all my advice, it is imperative to use your critical thinking and intuition to judge whether you feel the advice aligns with you and your personal desired outcomes and makes sense to you. In fact, that's the entire point of this book: to present all the reasons why the Triple-A Response® will help you.

To be clear, I think there are many wonderful practitioners out there, I really do. I just know some practitioners falsely claim they can help people with certain conditions when they can't, and this isn't just my experience. I've heard countless stories of people whose experiences are similar to mine. For this reason, it is my strong opinion that a large number of people struggling with OCD and anxiety are investing a ton of their time, energy, and money into products, programs, and inventions that won't provide results. In fact, in many cases, these people's symptoms are worsening as a result of these interventions—they likely would have been better off doing nothing at all.

OCD and Anxiety Recovery Is a Paradox

If you've taken the time to read this far, please read and memorize the following sentences: **Breaking out of the OCD & anxiety loop has nothing to do with eliminating your thoughts and feelings.** Instead, you need to shift your attention and energy to eliminating all the behaviors you are doing that are fueling the loop. Once you break the loop, the thoughts and feelings will decrease as a by-product.

I know this advice is probably not what you expected when you purchased this book. You likely bought this book because you wanted to learn how to get rid of intrusive thoughts and anxious feelings. And yet that's why this entire process is a complete paradox. It may even go against everything you've been told by other counselors. Right now, you may even be thinking, "Okay, this Matt guy is a little nuts." That's totally fine, but please hear me out.

The key to breaking out of the OCD & anxiety loop doesn't have anything to do with trying to make your thoughts go away or getting rid of your anxious feelings. On the contrary, the more you try to make the thoughts and feelings go away, the worse they will probably get. You may have been trying to accomplish this for a while, and the results should be clear: It doesn't work. If that path worked, you would be better by now.

The key is really understanding the four parts of the OCD & anxiety loop that we discussed in Chapter 2.

Here's a quick reminder:

1. You experience an intrusive thought.

2. This activates an uncomfortable feeling (the sympathetic nervous system).

3. You engage in a safety behavior.

4. That safety behavior produces a feeling of relief from the initial discomfort.

1
Past or Future-Based
Intrusive Thought

2
An Uncomfortable
Feeling

3
A Safety Behavior

4
A Feeling of
Short-Term Relief

Once you really get that your issue is a loop problem, not a thought or feeling problem, and ultimately that the loop is creating a lens that completely distorts your worldview, you can begin to understand that you really are not seeing things correctly and begin to shift your attention and energy into breaking the loop!

You do this by shifting your focus to your safety behaviors because that's the only thing you have control over. That's the truth, the whole truth, and nothing but the truth. That is the paradox of recovery. You break the OCD & anxiety loop when you stop engaging in all of your safety behaviors, mental and physical. That's it; it is the only way.

It is all about shifting your entire perspective—and in this OCD and anxiety recovery process, there are three key perspective changes you need to make. This chapter will talk through these three fundamental shifts you need to break the loop. Let's get started with the first one.

Shift No. 1: Your Intrusive Thoughts Are Not the Problem!

The first shift is letting go of the idea that you need to stop your intrusive thoughts. Let me back this up using some interesting studies from the 1980s and 1990s. Dr. Daniel Wegner, a social psychologist, conducted a series of studies on the act of thought suppression, obsessions, and psychological control. He presented most of his significant findings in his book *White Bears and Other Unwanted Thoughts*, in case you want to learn more.

In the studies, Daniel Wegner welcomed his test subjects into a room and asked them to track all of their thoughts for a specific period—I believe it was approximately ten minutes. During the study, there was one key instruction: Dr. Wegner specifically told the participants *not* to think about white bears. Wegner told each participant that if a white bear did, in fact, pop into their mind during the experiment, they were to record it (American Psychological Association, 2011).

Now, during the experiments, Wegner found that the participants kept experiencing thoughts about white bears, even though he'd explicitly told them not to. In fact, the participants in the study reported experiencing consistent thoughts of white bears during *and* after the study; some even reported dreams of white bears after the experiment was complete!

Okay, this is a lot of talk about white bears. What does this have to do with you? And what exactly is the point here? Wegner's research illustrates that suppressing a thought can cause it to rebound more strongly than if you weren't trying to suppress it at all. In other words, when you're telling yourself not to think about your intrusive thought, it comes up more often than if you were to just let it be. It is the *law of reversed effort* as explained by Emile Coue in his book *Self Mastery Through Conscious Autosuggestion*.

Unsurprisingly, Wegner wanted to explore this further. As his studies progressed, he discovered more and more about thought suppression. He began to hone his focus on attempting to answer the question, "Why is it so hard to get rid of unwanted thoughts?"

As his research progressed, he developed his *ironic processes theory*. He explained how two primary brain components are at odds when we attempt to avoid thinking about something. Simply put, one part of the brain actively alarms you if and when you experience a specific unwanted thought. Meanwhile, a second part of your brain constantly checks to ensure the unwanted thought hasn't appeared in your awareness. However, by trying not to think about a certain thought, you inadvertently create that thought in your mind, which, of course, sets off the alarm. This then causes the thought to pop up more and sets off the alarm again.

Try it for yourself: For the next sixty seconds, don't think of a blue tree.

See what I mean?

What Wegner demonstrated was the paradoxical effect of thought suppression (a common mental safety behavior). The more you try to avoid thinking a specific thought, whatever that thought may be, the more likely you are to experience it.

This exact dynamic is what happens when we try to solve OCD and anxiety as a thought problem. When we attempt to block, suppress, repress, replace, or eliminate our unwanted thoughts, these thoughts just show up more. As a result, we spend more effort trying to get rid of them. All those behaviors I just mentioned related to thoughts, including thought suppression, are massive safety behaviors.

They may be harder to notice than, say, washing your hands or switching the light on and off ten times, but they are still safety behaviors. The difference is this is a mental safety behavior, not a physical one. But we will go deeper into that in the next chapter.

So that's the first shift you need to make. Stop trying to control or fix your unwanted thoughts in any way, shape, or form. It doesn't matter what they are saying; it's not your business.

You might be thinking, "WAIT A MINUTE! What do you mean it's not my business? These are my thoughts—of course, they are my business." Well, in chapter 6, I will introduce the idea of shifting into a higher level of consciousness.

I promise this will make more sense in a little bit. But please don't skip ahead—you're going to need to do these shifts first, so trust the process!

The next shift is related to your feelings.

Shift No. 2: It's OK to Feel Feelings!

When people hear about OCD and anxiety, the vast majority view this experience as something they need to get rid of. Like some weird, abnormal growth on your body. They want to amputate it and be rid of it. (I know, great visual, huh?)

I believe one of the primary reasons people want to get rid of anxiety so badly is simply because they think that feeling anything other than happy is abnormal. But let's challenge that for a second. Is anxiety really abnormal? Stress is a normal response to challenges we face in life. Challenges are expected; therefore, stress is normal.

As we discussed last chapter, psychological stress is when our minds attempt to predict possible challenges and resolve them, and as we know, this doesn't work out very well. The *Diagnostic and Statistical Manual of Psychiatric Disorders* (*DSM*) categorizes these different manifestations of psychological stress as different mental health disorders.

Now, while I believe that a diagnosis can be extremely helpful in directing someone to a proper course of treatment, the biggest misconception most people have is that the presence of anxiety in the body indicates a disorder. That couldn't be farther from the truth. It is actually the resistance to the anxiety itself that causes people to engage in safety behaviors. And when a person engages in safety behaviors throughout the day to avoid anxiety, it *creates* disorder in their life. However, if people are taught to believe that anxiety is not normal, it makes sense that they would try to get rid of it, and therein lies the problem.

Whenever I give a presentation, I try and combat this assumption that anxiety is a problem right away. I usually ask the audience, "How many people in this room have felt anxious?" Every time, without fail, every hand in the room goes up. So the question becomes, "How can anxiety be abnormal if everyone experiences it?" Either we all have mental health disorders, or we are all mislabeling a totally normal experience as a disorder.

MATT'S TINFOIL HAT MOMENT

Okay, I have these moments from time to time throughout the book because I can't help myself. If you don't like these personal shares, just skip over them. But if we look at the question, "Why would we pathologize a totally normal human experience like anxiety?" and then we take a peek behind the big pharma curtain, it just so happens that some organizations in our world massively profit from convincing a bunch of people that a normal experience is abnormal. Through this misconception, these organizations are able to create and sell certain products that reduce the symptoms while never addressing the behavioral cause. This potentially creates a scenario for a person to be dependent on the product and as a result creates lifelong reoccurring customers and higher profits. Just sayin'. Okay, enough of that. Back to the book.

We can debate this idea, but I choose to believe that anxiety is an entirely normal experience. However, as I said, if we believe that anxiety is abnormal, it causes us to resist the experience.

This makes us do a bunch of different behaviors to remove or control anxiety.

Just like intrusive thoughts, this creates a paradoxical experience through the law of reversed effort, where we experience more anxiety. As Carl Jung describes in his book, *The Structure and Dynamics of the Psyche*, whatever you resist, persists.

Therefore, the presence of anxiety in the body does not indicate a disorder. The attempt to eliminate and control anxious feelings by performing safety behaviors is what creates a persistent experience of anxiety. And continuous engagement in safety behaviors creates disorder in a person's life. The feeling isn't at fault here.

This distinction is vital to your success. It's so important that it's worth repeating multiple times in this section and throughout the book.

So my official stance is the feeling of anxiety is not a disorder, but because we believe it's a problem, we engage in a bunch of behaviors to get rid of or control the anxious feelings, thereby creating disorder in our lives.

You see, the more we try to fight our unwanted thoughts and anxious feelings by performing safety behaviors, the more frequently and intensely they arise. Think about trying to push a beach ball underwater. You can push that ball down all you want, but as soon as you let go, it will bounce right back up to the surface.

Feelings are just like this—you can try to keep them under the surface, but not for long. They'll find their way up in some way, shape, or form.

The truth is, feelings are normal. We humans have a whole spectrum of emotions, and feeling these emotions is a natural human process. Feeling our feelings is what helps the nervous system metabolize them. In fact, it's an essential part of our health. There is fascinating work published on the connection between emotional suppression and disease if you wish to dive deeper. For the purpose of this book, just remember that healing comes through feeling. When it comes to anxiety (and our other emotions), we must be willing to embrace it when it comes to the surface.

So, this is the second shift: Stop directing your energy toward trying to get rid of your anxiety. Your feelings are normal and meant to be felt—it's OK to feel whatever you are feeling.

So, if you shouldn't eliminate your thoughts or feelings, what should you be focusing on?

This brings us to our third and final shift: stopping your safety behaviors.

Shift No. 3: Stop Doing Your Safety Behaviors!

The third shift is plain and simple—to direct your energy and attention toward stopping your safety behaviors. This is the only way to truly break the OCD & anxiety loop. It's the only thing that can stop the loop from spinning because it's the only thing you actually have control over.

I want to acknowledge something real quick. Safety behaviors *do* work for combating intrusive thoughts and anxious feelings. They are a quick way to relieve the built-up pressure of thoughts and feelings. If they didn't work, we wouldn't do them. The problem is that safety behaviors never work in the long term. They merely suppress the uncomfortable thoughts and feelings for a little while.

They're a short-term solution. Just when you feel like your safety behavior has worked magic, the pressure quickly accumulates again. This means you'll have to continue engaging in more safety behaviors, which will eventually create a long-term problem. That's why we had to make those first two shifts before we got here.

One metaphor I like to use when discussing the OCD & anxiety loop is pressure gauges and release valves. You have a thought gauge, a feeling gauge, and a behavior valve, and they all influence each other. When the pressure in the thought gauge goes up, it triggers the pressure in the feeling gauge to go up, and when you pull the behavior release level, it causes the thought and feeling gauge to go down.

That's what it's like with the OCD & anxiety loop. The thoughts pop up and bring about an uncomfortable feeling that pushes you to take action. So you engage in the safety behavior, which temporarily relieves you of the discomfort. Then the thought comes back again, so you pull the behavior valve again, and again, and again.

Let's use this in a real-world example, shall we? Let's pretend that you've been pulling this behavior release valve day after day for a long time. Then someone tells you that the thought and feeling gauges have their own built-in regulation system and will automatically go down on their own over time. So all you have to do is sit tight and do nothing. You are actually preventing this automatic regulation system from kicking in because you keep pulling this release valve.

So you decide to follow this advice. Instead of focusing on controlling the thought and feeling gauges, you hone in on one task, not pulling the behavior valve—effectively, you do nothing.

Instead, you just watch as the pressure increases and trust that the system will regulate itself. At this point, you likely feel a lot of discomfort and uncertainty, especially the first few times you try it. Why? Because you've spent so much time regulating the thought and feeling gauge yourself with the behavior valve, it feels like just "doing nothing" will lead to something terrible happening. The first time you do this, it is very intense. However, over time, you begin to notice that the pressure in the thought and feeling gauges begins to go down on its own.

Changing the way you view the situation and trusting the system allows the pressure to increase and decrease without intervening. You begin to trust that the pressure is nothing to fear. It's an imagined threat.

In the same way, by repositioning your focus to your safety behaviors, we begin to target the only thing we're in control of— the thing that will break this debilitating OCD & anxiety loop. I spent a long time trying to control everything outside my control. But what I learned, after many years, is that you can't control your thoughts or feelings; they just come up! The only thing you have absolute control over is your behavior. So that is where you need to place your attention and energy.

An interesting thing happens once we start refraining from safety behaviors. Sure, our thoughts and feelings will continue to pop up initially when we stop engaging in safety behaviors, which can be scary. But if we stick with this, we begin to see that they become less frequent with time. And why is this? Because we're no longer reinforcing them. Remember that whole idea of conditioning we discussed earlier?

By saying, "Hey, it's OK if you come up to the surface; I'll just let you pass in your own time without trying to control you," you recognize that your body and mind are reacting to an imagined threat, not a real one. In doing so, your unwanted thoughts and feelings lose weight. You stop reinforcing them and begin to understand that they are normal and not dangerous.

We call this process *habituation*. Habitation is the gradual decline of your physical and mental responses through repeated exposure to a specific stimulus (van Hout and Emmelkamp, 2002). For example, you might have the sexiest spouse on the planet, the nicest house on the block, or the coolest car, but over time, the initial spike of pride, warmth, excitement, etc. you felt when these things came into your life will get lower and lower as you get used to the idea of having them. You habituate. The same holds true with anxiety—when you stop engaging in your safety behaviors, you're proving to your nervous system that you have no need to fear the thing that's causing you stress and anxiety.

This doesn't mean ignoring your intrusive thoughts or anxious feelings altogether. You are aware they are there and acknowledge their presence, but you do nothing to get rid of them. You coexist with them as you would an annoying house guest—you wait for them to leave on their own accord. When you do this repeatedly, you recondition your brain and nervous system to recognize that these thoughts and feelings aren't dangerous. And gradually, your mind and body realize that there was literally no need to be afraid in the first place and that your safety behaviors weren't keeping you safe because there was no real threat to begin with—it was a perceived threat.

This moves us onto Exposure and Response Prevention, one of the primary modalities we will be building upon throughout this process of breaking out of your OCD & anxiety loop.

Exposure and Response Prevention

If you've researched OCD and anxiety treatment, you likely have read or heard something about Exposure and Response Prevention (ERP). If you're new to this concept, though, don't fret! It's pretty easy to understand. Let's break it down! The *exposure* part refers to facing your fear by **exposing** yourself to the thought/object/situation/person causing you stress. The *response prevention* part means you **prevent** yourself from **responding** to the stressful stimuli with a safety behavior.

So to put it very simply, ERP is facing your fears without engaging in safety behaviors.

Let's bring back our fear of contamination example to go deeper into this concept. Remember the person who would experience a fear of contamination after they touched a doorknob? The act of touching the doorknob is the external trigger, and the internal triggers begin going off with all those what-if thoughts like, "What if I get AIDS?" This, in turn, sets off their stress response.

So in this scenario, both the external trigger of touching a doorknob and the internal trigger, the what-if thoughts, are forms of exposure. Some people experience more external triggers, and other people experience more internal triggers—it really depends on the individual's experience. But both experiences are examples of exposures because they activate the stress response.

Once the stress response is activated, the brain and body scream at the person to do some type of safety behavior to mitigate the potential threat. This could be a physical safety behavior (e.g., washing their hands, researching AIDS on the internet, or calling their doctor for reassurance), or it could be a mental safety behavior (e.g., reassuring themselves, trying to suppress the scary thoughts, or ruminating about the contamination experience).

But say this person decided to practice ERP in this heightened state—they choose to stay with the anxiety and prevent themselves from engaging in *any* safety behavior. They avoid any response that would immediately shift them out of the anxious state. They allow the anxious thoughts and uncomfortable feelings to surface and then dissipate on their own accord. Eventually, their stress response returns to baseline, and they go about their day. That is what Exposure and Response Prevention is.

You see, by not engaging in the behaviors, the brain is forced to assess, "Is this situation actually dangerous?" A mental transformation (habituation) then occurs when they see, through repeated exposure, that the stimulus had no dangerous or threatening outcome—it was safe. Then, instead of perceiving this stimulus as a threat, it becomes an everyday experience. The individual can now touch a doorknob, and the alarm bells won't go off in their head because they have had consistent proof that it won't cause them harm.

You see, if you continue engaging in your safety behaviors, your brain never gets the opportunity to challenge the assumption that the feared stimulus is dangerous. You'll forever be fearful of that particular thought, object, person, or situation. The loop will just keep spinning. Or you can choose to change your ways and rewire your brain so that this fearful stimulus no longer triggers you, using ERP.

Of course, while this process sounds simple, it's not easy! It takes hard work. It also requires courage, strength, and perseverance, especially when you've been battling these fears for a long time. However, it can be done, regardless of the severity or duration of your OCD and anxious thoughts. You just have to be prepared to ride the wave of anxiety whenever it pops up. Once you begin engaging in ERP consistently, you're on the path to rewiring your brain to operate in a much healthier way.

Neuroplasticity & Rewiring the Brain

"Can I really rewire my brain," you ask?

Well, in my opinion, no one explains this better than Dr. Jeffrey Schwartz and Dr. Rebecca Gladding. In their book *You Are Not Your Brain,* they talk at length about this idea of neuroplasticity and the brain's power to heal and rewire. They state in the book that our brain's ability to do this is rooted in Hebb's law and the quantum Zeno effect.

In case you are wondering . . . you *can* rewire your brain! When I first read about neuroplasticity, Hebb's law, and the quantum Zeno effect, I felt overwhelmed because they were way out of my element. So it's OK if you feel that way too.

I hated any topics even marginally related to science in school. These ideas often feel far out of my league. Luckily, you don't need to understand this for it to work. Do you understand how your body digests food or heals a cut on your knee or hand? I sure don't. But my body seems to do it anyway. It's the same principle here.

Let's be very clear—I am in no way a neuroscientist, nor do I want to be. But I found these concepts helpful in my own recovery, and I hope you will too. I am going to attempt to explain this at an elementary level in this book, and if you want to geek out on these topics, by all means, go ahead—I recommend starting with Dr. Schwartz's work.

Anyway, Hebb's Law basically states that "neurons that fire together, wire together." Essentially, this means that your brain activates particular neurons when you perform specific behavior patterns. Over time, when you continue this behavior pattern, the connection between these neurons strengthens.

This is a highly beneficial system, but unfortunately, it can work against us. When you perform a safety behavior for the first time, especially to alleviate an uncomfortable feeling, you create a new neural connection. This connection strengthens as you continue to engage in this behavior whenever you experience this uncomfortable feeling. Over time, this circuit can become so strong that you do your safety behaviors almost without thinking about them, and that's because you've reinforced the neural connections through repetition.

But the good news is what can be done can always be undone—our neural pathways change all the time. The myth that you are stuck with the brain you have has been debunked. Your brain is constantly learning and evolving with everything you do, no matter how old you are. Just because your neural pathway for your safety behaviors is strong now doesn't mean it will be forever. By preventing yourself from engaging in your safety behaviors now, you can weaken this connection and, in doing so, begin to form healthier connections at a cellular level.

Dr. Schwartz and Dr. Gladding offer a great analogy for neuroplasticity—they simply talk about walking on a new hiking trail. Let me explain it. There's a hiker who goes on the same hiking trail every day, but he's not particularly happy with this trail because he doesn't like the views. The hiker is looking to get closer to the most scenic areas, and he can see that off the track, there are already some patches of dirt that have been cleared of all the brush. He just has to clear a path between the patches of dirt to form a new trail.

So he decides to venture off the path and create a new trail for himself. At first, he struggles to see where he's going, as the path isn't formed—he has to step over all the brush and plants. He keeps walking this new path day after day. And slowly, over time, the overgrowth is trampled down, and the new path is easy to walk along. He knows where he's going because he's now walked the trail many times. What's more, other hikers have now also ditched the old route and have started using this new one!

Here's the really interesting part: Since all the hikers now use this new path, gradually, the old path becomes overgrown because there's no one walking on it. The new scenic trail is now the preferred and only route. See the power of that?

To be clear, in this metaphor, the scenic route's cleared patches of dirt are the neurons that are yet to form a connection. The hiker is the neurotransmitter. When the hiker starts to walk along the scenic way, this is equivalent to performing a new behavior pattern. It begins to create links between the cleared patches of dirt (or the neurons). Gradually, this connection strengthens because it's readily used by other hikers (or neurotransmitters). And hence, a new path is created, a new link is formed, and the old path begins to weaken.

Studies and brain scans show that you can literally create physical changes within your brain through Exposure and Response Prevention and habituation (Simpson and Hazel, 2019; Saxena et al., 2008). Even someone with the most severe panic reaction to a specific stimulus can reduce it significantly. The capability to do this doesn't depend on age, gender, race, or any other demographic quality. You can rewire your brain regardless of how often you have intrusive thoughts or how long they've been plaguing your life. And, yes, this applies to you and your exact situation too. You just need to stop engaging in your safety behaviors—all of them. Your safety behaviors have to be reduced to zero.

Again, I stress that while this sounds simple, it's not easy. It requires persistence and will most likely cause significant anxiety to begin with. That's why we personally guide our clients through this process in my Taking Back Control Program and my group coaching and individual coaching programs. You can learn more about those at **www.restoredminds.com/tbc**.

What's more, some safety behaviors are harder to stop than others. For example, you can tell yourself not to wash your hands or ask others for reassurance. But how do you stop mental behaviors like suppressing or replacing thoughts, analyzing, ruminating, and worrying? These are a little trickier to tackle. However, it can still be done with the right strategy and perspective. Meet me in chapter 5, where you can begin to identify your own mental safety behaviors.

Chapter Five
Mental Safety Behaviors

*"I've suffered a great many catastrophes in my life.
Most of them never happened."*

Mark Twain

I've had the opportunity to learn a lot through my time working with people who struggle with OCD and anxiety. Along the road, I've also had the chance to reflect on and study my own journey to recovery. This is how I know that of all the knowledge and insights I've gained throughout this time, perhaps none is more important than this—**mental safety behaviors are one of the (if not the) primary reason people stay stuck in the OCD & anxiety loop.** I fully believe mental safety behaviors are the most misunderstood and overlooked aspects of breaking free from OCD and anxiety. You see, many people engage in mental safety behaviors without even realizing they're doing it. Because of this, stopping is much more difficult.

To kick off this chapter, I want to share a story with you. When I was really stuck in the OCD and anxiety lens, I did several mental safety behaviors, such as thought suppression, thought blocking, replacing bad thoughts with good thoughts, silent prayer, mental rumination, and reviewing and analyzing my past. And while I was able to identify my physical safety behaviors really well, my mental safety behaviors went unnoticed and unaddressed. No one even suggested to me that they were a problem. Not for years! I thought everyone did these things, like eating or breathing. It was a strange idea when it was finally suggested to me that it was unhealthy to be in my head all day.

When I was really stuck, I spent most of my day engaging in mental safety behaviors. In fact, I can recall one occasion when I was sitting in a college lecture, and the class began, and the class ended, and I couldn't tell you one thing that had been taught by the professor. I was so in my own head, analyzing and ruminating, that I hadn't comprehended a word the professor had said.

I'm sharing this story with you because I've seen many people experience something similar on their own journey. For the majority of my clients, when they finally learn about mental behaviors, their entire journey changes. We talked briefly about mental safety behaviors in Chapter 2. Here, we'll explore how mental safety behaviors feed into the loop, just like physical safety behaviors. We'll also go into more detail about the different kinds of safety behaviors many people perform in their heads. That way, you can begin identifying which ones you might be performing. This is the next step to breaking out of the loop.

How Mental Safety Behaviors Feed the Loop

It is essential for your recovery to know, and I haven't really specified this to this point, that performing *any* safety behavior will create the OCD & anxiety loop, whatever it is. Your safety behavior could be washing your hands, turning a light switch on and off ten times, avoiding grocery stores, smoking weed, drinking alcohol, purging after a meal, or things like rumination and mentally analyzing. Whatever the safety behavior, it will feed the loop. They all work in the same way.

So, what makes a behavior a safety behavior? Well, it all comes down to why you engage in the behavior. Drinking alcohol can be a safety behavior for one person and a regular activity for another. It's about whether the behavior creates fast relief from an internal emotional discomfort. Any action that temporarily relieves an intrusive thought is a safety behavior. Therefore, anything that alleviates anxiety or unwanted thoughts feeds the OCD & anxiety loop.

That's why our goal is to eliminate *all s*afety behaviors. We need to reduce that behavior gauge to zero. This is where a lot of people veer off course. They eliminate their physical safety behaviors because they're easier to recognize. So they successfully stop performing them and hope their unwanted thoughts and feelings reduce. But they, often unknowingly, keep doing their mental safety behaviors, so they never achieve habituation.

Even though they stopped their physical safety behaviors, their loop never breaks because they are still engaging in safety behaviors. Then they take the really bad step of concluding that Exposure and Response Prevention "doesn't work for me." They assume they have a special case—that they are the exception, not the rule.

Let me address this head-on. You are the rule, not the exception! This will work for you. If you haven't had success to this point, it is most likely because you are engaging in behaviors that reinforce the loop without realizing it. The truth is, the only way the OCD & anxiety loop will stop spinning is if you eliminate all of your safety behaviors.

To better illustrate mental safety behaviors, I'll use an example of a man I once worked with. This man, we'll call him Simon, was afraid of flying. He had catastrophic thoughts whenever he knew he would have to fly somewhere. He would envision the plane crashing or something terrible happening. Now, unfortunately for Simon, traveling was a requirement for his work, so he often found himself in this situation.

In the upcoming days before a flight, Simon's mind was flooded with plane-related what-if thoughts. It began with thoughts like, "What if the plane crashes?" and spiraled from there, as we know it does. Some of the what-if thoughts plaguing him were as follows:

- "What if something happens to me and my family is left without me?"
- "What if my life insurance doesn't pay out?"
- "What if they can't afford to pay for the house?"
- "What if they end up homeless?"
- "What if my wife can't afford to send our kids to college?"

His mind ran on this kind of tangent week after week. Eventually, when he realized these what-if thoughts were significantly impacting his life, he sought help in my Taking Back Control Program. Quickly, he recognized that it was a combination of physical and mental safety behaviors reinforcing his OCD & anxiety loop. So, together, we did a behavior inventory—an essential part of the program. It involves identifying all of the safety behaviors you engage in.

We focused on all of Simon's physical safety behaviors, to begin with. He had no problem identifying these. He told me that he wears his lucky jacket, hat, and shoes every time he flies. He has a special cocktail before he boards the plane, says his Rosaries, and tries to always upgrade to the exit row when he gets on the plane, so he can be the first one out of the plane in the event of an emergency. We won't get into the fact that people in the exit row are supposed to help other passengers exit the plane first because, for the people on the flight with Simon, that simply wasn't going to happen (at least not at that point in his life).

Now, each of these behaviors provided a certain level of relief; that's how we knew they were safety behaviors. And, of course, we knew that none of Simon's behaviors caused the plane to land safely, so we systematically began removing these. He purposefully didn't wear his lucky clothing, drank a different drink, didn't say his Rosaries, and chose an "unsafe" row on the plane. As he did this, the plane still landed safely when he flew. This reinforced the fact in his mind that these behaviors weren't actually keeping him safe.

But as we have discussed, stopping only his physical safety behaviors wasn't enough. To ensure we really broke the loop, we also had to get rid of his mental safety behaviors.

Identifying his mental safety behaviors was more challenging. This process is often more tricky because these actions tend to sit just on the fringe of our conscious awareness; they're not as apparent as physical behaviors. We really had to get honest about everything he was doing mentally to protect himself from his fear of flying. We figured out that he was mentally reassuring and distracting himself several days before the flight, ruminating over thoughts about what would happen if he died, attempting to block and suppress scary thoughts, and several other mental behaviors.

It wasn't until we began eliminating all the mental safety behaviors that Simon really saw the benefits of the Exposure and Response Prevention process.

Now it's time for you to identify your own mental safety behaviors. Below, there's a breakdown of some of the most common mental safety behaviors many people engage in.

Common Mental Safety Behaviors

We can do many mental safety behaviors to relieve anxious feelings and intrusive thoughts. Here is a breakdown of the most common ones I encounter:

- Mental review/mental analyzing
- Rumination
- Mental reassurance
- Mental checking/scanning
- Distraction
- Thought suppression
- Thought replacement
- Silent prayer
- Counting
- Mentally repeating words/phrases

Before I go on, it's important to say that these are not the only mental safety behaviors. These are just broad categories that have resonated with many of my clients and other people wrestling with OCD and anxiety. Any psychological behavior that relieves anxiety or intrusive thoughts could be classified as a mental safety behavior.

Okay, let's dive into it.

Mental Review/Mental Analyzing

When someone experiences anxiety, it is usually followed by the belief that some type of problem needs to be solved. Mental review and analyzing are mental safety behaviors that people use to try to solve the perceived problems in their minds.

This particular mental safety behavior operates off two false premises:

1. There is a real dilemma that you must solve when anxiety is generally rooted in a past or future possible scenario.

2. When you worry about or analyze something, you are actually "doing something" that will resolve the issue.

In actuality, the possible scenario doesn't really exist, so all that is happening is that you are lost in your head and distracted from the present moment.

Rumination

Rumination means to ponder or think deeply about something. The root word *ruminant* actually refers to how cows chew, swallow, and then regurgitate food and chew it again. Cows do this because it increases their nutritional intake and improves digestion.

So effectively, when you ruminate about something, think of it like chewing on a thought over and over. People can ruminate about intrusive thoughts or possible scenarios in an attempt to reduce the discomfort they are experiencing. And, of course, rumination does make us feel better, even if it's only for a few moments, because it creates the illusion that we are "doing something" about the problem.

Mental Reassurance

Mental reassurance is pretty straightforward. You're mentally reassuring yourself when you try to make yourself feel better by telling yourself it will be OK, that you will be fine, and so on. For it to be mental reassurance rather than plain old reassurance, it needs to be happening inside your head—you're not saying it verbally.

For example, if you have a fear of contamination, this could be telling yourself (in your head), "I'm actually OK; I don't have AIDS," again and again after you encounter an external trigger, like touching a doorknob. This reassurance may make you feel better in the short term, but it reinforces the loop because it encourages you to treat the situation as dangerous in the future.

Mental Checking/Scanning

Mental checking and scanning are when you internally check or scan your body for something. This could be a body scan to see if something is out of the ordinary for health anxiety. It could be checking to see if you were sexually aroused by something. It could be checking for the presence of anxiety or intrusive thoughts.

Again, mental checking reinforces the idea that your worries about this intrusive thought are valid, further spinning the loop.

Distraction

Distraction is another common mental safety behavior. It involves thinking about or doing something else to get rid of intrusive thoughts or anxious feelings.

By attempting to distract ourselves, we're avoiding our thoughts and feelings. Many people with OCD and anxiety will flood themselves with external stimuli (i.e., music, podcasts, television, social gatherings, working out, etc.).

Again, it's not that these things are bad—it's all about the context of why you are doing them. If you use these things or anything else to distract yourself from your uncomfortable thoughts and feelings, it reinforces the idea these are dangerous.

Distractions provide temporary relief, but our unwanted ideas are still there, under the surface, unaddressed.

Thought Suppression/Blocking

Thought suppression refers to when you try to block or eliminate an intrusive thought when it pops up. This brings us back to Dr. Wegner's studies and the ironic process discussed in the previous chapter.

But, as I explained in chapter 4, thought suppression only serves to further reinforce the loop, as it makes you experience the intrusive thought more and more.

Thought Replacement

Thought replacement involves swapping out an intrusive thought for a "safe" or "good" thought. This has a similar effect to thought suppression, ending in a constant battle between you and your thoughts. And even if you prefer thinking about the "good thought," it just reinforces the idea that the "bad thought" you're experiencing is a threatening situation.

Silent Prayer

Okay, we are going to move into controversial waters here. So let me clarify something—prayer isn't bad. In fact, I'd personally argue prayer is good—prayer is an integral part of my personal life. I totally believe in the power of prayer.

With that being said, it is vital to distinguish the intention behind using prayer when it comes to OCD and anxiety. If you are praying as an expression of your faith, then, of course, carry on! But if you're praying to instantly make yourself feel better about an obsession or unwanted thought, prayer is acting as a safety behavior and will gradually worsen your anxiety with repetition.

By silently praying to scrap the intrusive thoughts or anxiety, you're training your brain to believe that the unwanted thoughts and anxiety are actually dangerous. After all, if something's not dangerous, why would you need to pray for an intervention?

However, no intervention needs to take place. Think of a young child praying for God to protect him from the monster under his bed. Sure, it may make him feel better, but nothing needs to happen because there never was a monster under the bed. The problem is that when nothing happens to the child, it reinforces the idea that God saved him from the monster when, in actuality, there was no monster.

So praying against intrusive thoughts and anxiety will perpetuate the exact thoughts and feelings you don't want, and you'll wind up spending hours of your day praying, just like I was.

Counting

This is one of the most well-known OCD and anxiety mental safety behaviors. A great example is the movie *As Good as It Gets*. The movie depicts Melvin Udall (played by Jack Nicholson) turning lights on and off and flipping the latch on the door a precise number of times. Melvin (as well as many others struggling with OCD and anxiety) does this because he believes it's a safe number.

I remember a young girl who believed that she had to count to any number she saw; otherwise, her parents would be in danger. So every number she saw, she stopped and silently counted to whatever number was in front of her to prevent something terrible from happening to her parents. Just take a second and imagine her experience walking down a school hallway . . . room 101, room 103, room 105. You get the idea.

As with all mental safety behaviors, counting creates a false connection where you believe the act of counting prevents a negative outcome. In this scenario, the young girl counted because she thought this was the only way to protect her parents. When, in truth, her parents were never in danger.

Another way counting presents in OCD and anxiety is to distract yourself from intrusive thoughts. In this instance, counting and distraction are used in unison to ease the discomfort caused by unwanted ideas.

Repeating Words/Phrases

This is when you repeat words or phrases in your head to relieve yourself of a fearful or anxious feeling or to counteract intrusive thoughts. Repeating words and phrases may reassure you that you're safe or could distract you from thinking about an unwanted idea.

But don't be fooled. This act is a safety behavior because it tells your brain that the feelings/intrusive thoughts are something you need to protect yourself against.

I hope you see the trend here and understand that it is all about the intention behind the behavior, not the behavior itself. Moreover, the mental safety behaviors I described above are just some of the most common ones I see when working with people.

Final Note

The real takeaway of this chapter is that mental safety behaviors need to be removed, just like physical safety behaviors, in order for you to get better. And unless you are aware of them, there's a very high probability you'll continue engaging in them without even realizing it.

If you've been trying Exposure and Response Prevention and haven't experienced habituation, are you sure you've eliminated *all* of your safety behaviors? If not, you aren't doing ERP fully. You are engaging in exposure, for sure, but then you're using your safety behaviors. That's what's causing the OCD & anxiety loop to keep going.

You now understand your mental safety behaviors. The next piece of the puzzle is understanding the strategy for breaking out of the loop. In order to do this, we must first understand the concept of different levels of consciousness. Join me in the next chapter, where we dive into this.

CHAPTER SIX

A Higher Level of Consciousness

"The moment you become aware of the ego in you, it is strictly speaking no longer the ego, but just an old, conditioned mind-pattern. Ego implies unawareness. Awareness and ego cannot coexist."

Eckhart Tolle

Many people that wrestle with OCD and anxiety find themselves bouncing around from book to book, program to program, and therapist to therapist. Why? Because they are looking for that magic pill or special tool to get rid of their intrusive thoughts and anxiety. I know this because I was one of them.

There's a fundamental problem with this approach. Essentially, you're trying to solve the problem of OCD and anxiety by using specific tools from the same level of consciousness that created the problem in the first place. Along with the mental safety behaviors we covered in the last chapter, this is the most common barrier to success that I see people encounter—I fell into this trap for many years on my journey. This is why I want to discuss this concept before we move forward.

Before we dive into the Triple-A Response®, let's get to know the fundamental concept of consciousness, because the Triple-A Response® will only work if implemented from a higher level of consciousness. As Albert Einstein famously said, "A problem can't be solved from the same level of consciousness that created it." This holds true for OCD and anxiety as well. You can't solve a thought problem by thinking about it more.

Now I know there will probably be many people who purchase this book and skip to the chapters on the Triple-A Response®. But by skipping over this one concept of consciousness, they will very likely experience a great deal of frustration when they try to implement the Triple-A Response® in their life. Luckily, that's not you, because you are reading this right now. Thank you for not skipping ahead.

I will repeat this one more time because I can't stress the importance of this enough. The Triple-A Response® will only be effective if you apply it from a higher level of consciousness.

Okay, so what is consciousness? I googled the definition, and it read, "The state or condition of being conscious." Hmm, thanks for that one, Google. I really dislike when people use the word you're trying to define in the definition. Since I didn't find that very helpful, I guessed you wouldn't either, so I decided to dig a little deeper.

Currently, my favorite definition of consciousness is by John Randolph Price in his book *Nothing Is Too Good to Be True*. In the book, Price defined consciousness as simply "having **awareness**, **understanding**, and **knowledge** about any particular aspect of life." Let's use a simple example, like multiplication tables, to explain this. You are probably *aware* that multiplication tables exist. You probably *understand* what they are, and you likely possess the *knowledge* of how to apply them when necessary.

Therefore, by this definition, you possess a high level of consciousness regarding multiplication tables. You are aware of them, understand them, and know how to apply them. Therefore, you are conscious of them.

But what do I mean when I talk about *self-consciousness* and *your consciousness*? And what does it mean when I talk about the levels of consciousness? All great questions! Let's break it down.

The suffix *-ness* means to "be in a state of." For example, *happiness* means "being in a state where you are happy." Therefore, *consciousness* means "being in a state where you are aware, understand, and know some particular aspect of life."

Let's move to the idea of *self-consciousness*, because this is a common term that most people can relate to—we are talking about the *small self* here, and I will elaborate on this idea later. Now when we discuss the concept of *self-consciousness*, all it really means is "to be in a state where you are aware, know, and understand yourself." But remember how I said you have different levels of consciousness?

Usually when we discuss the idea of someone who is self-conscious (small self), your mind probably immediately jumps to someone you know who is very anxious and neurotic. And usually means someone who is overly aware of and concerned with how they present to others and other people's opinions of them. While this is technically self-consciousness, it is a low level of self-consciousness.

This level of consciousness is often referred to as the *ego* or the *small self*. Your ego is simply your current self-concept developed by your mind. It is your mind's attempt to understand you. Your ego is built upon all your current labels and identities and heavily influenced by the environment in which you were raised. Your ego presents as the voice that is constantly talking in your mind. You know that voice that you hear all day? Your ego is judging everything that's happening, labeling things as good or bad, and attempting to keep you safe by predicting all these terrible things that can happen to you in the future.

So when we see someone who is self-conscious, we are actually saying that they are ego-conscious, meaning they are in a state where they are aware, understand, and know themselves to be the ego. They believe that they are actually this voice in their head. Therefore, in this level of consciousness, whatever the voice says, the person assumes this must actually be true, and they generally follow along with the direction of the voice in the mind.

Now, I'm not going to do a deep dive into explaining the ego in this book. The only thing I want you to understand is that the ego exists, and when we live from a place of ego-consciousness, we are aware, understand, and know ourselves as the ego. And this is one of the lowest levels of consciousness we can operate from. This state of consciousness generally leads us to function very reactively and willfully.

Now don't get upset about this; most of the people on this planet live from this state of consciousness and aren't even aware of an alternative way of living, or dare I say, they are not conscious of an alternative. And don't buy into the "woke culture" currently being promoted in our society, which proclaims to be operating from a higher level of thinking.

So now that we understand ego-consciousness, let's move to the idea of living from different levels of consciousness. When we talk about consciousness, we are talking about your state of awareness, understanding, and knowledge of yourself.

And if there are higher states of consciousness available to you and you aren't the ego, then the question is, who are you? We could probably spend a whole book on this idea and barely scratch the surface. Most people mistakenly think they know the answer to this question. But do me a favor and sit with this question for a minute.

If I asked you, "Who are you?" you might be inclined to answer with a specific label, for instance, your name ... In my case, it would be, "I am Matt." But is that true? Can't I legally change my name to Tom, Mike, Tree, or whatever I want? Would I actually change at all if I changed my name (or any labels)? No, probably not.

What if they removed the letter *M* from the English alphabet? Would I just be Att? Would I instantly lose part of myself? No, probably not.

So if you aren't a name or any other label, you might be inclined to answer that you are your body. Or maybe you want to sound more sophisticated (as the ego often does) and say, "I am the biological organism that occupies this physical space."

Oh, that's an excellent answer. But wait a minute, doesn't your body constantly change? I looked in the mirror when I was ten, and the image was totally different from when I looked at a mirror this morning at thirty-five. Am *I* really changing that significantly all the time? What if I suddenly lost my arms and legs? Would I lose a large portion of myself? No, probably not.

Or, as we discussed earlier, you might be inclined to answer that you are your mind. But wait, don't your thoughts change all the time? Don't you have random thoughts that pop up automatically? And can't you actually create specific thoughts on command? What about dreams? When you have dreams, are the dreams really who you are?

Here's a fascinating question. If your mind ceased functioning— if it was just still and quiet—would that mean you stopped existing? No, of course not. You would still be there.

I could go on here, but my point is that this is a tougher question to answer than you might assume. It's no wonder Socrates, the father of modern philosophy, taught with great importance the concept of "know thyself."

So what's the answer? Who are you? Well, to share my current view, I would draw mainly from the work of teachers like Michael Singer and Eckhart Tolle. To put it simply, you are the awareness. You are the one inside that is aware of what is happening. You are the one who hears the thoughts in your head; you are not the thoughts themselves. You are the one who is aware of and watches your dreams; you are not the dreams themselves. You are the one who notices the feelings in your body; you are not the feelings themselves. Your internal and external experiences change all the time, but you are the consistent awareness of it all.

This is the shift into a new level of consciousness, a state where you develop a new awareness, understanding, and knowledge of who you actually are. This is the shift into what Michael Singer calls "witness consciousness" (Singer, 2020). Witness consciousness means living in a state where you are aware, understand, and know yourself as the witness inside. Some call it the observing self or the higher self. Some might even go as far as to call it the spirit or soul.

Ultimately, it doesn't matter what you call it because you would just be creating another label. The reality is that you (the awareness) are constantly in a state of subject-object awareness, meaning you are the subject, and what you are aware of are the objects. And since there is a subject-object relationship, you cannot be the same thing you are aware of.

For instance, when you watch television, you know you are not the television; you are the one watching the television. Even deeper, you are the one who is aware that you are watching television. The television is the object, and you are the subject, aware that you are watching it. The same holds true with your internal experiences. You are not your thoughts and feelings; you are the complete, separate, and constant awareness that is aware of them. Your body, thoughts, and feelings change constantly, but you are the continual awareness behind it all. You have always been there, and you will always be there.

It's OK if you aren't fully grasping this right now—it's a lot to take in. It truly is an entirely new way of understanding and conceptualizing yourself. But it is so important because when you shift your self-consciousness from ego-consciousness to awareness-consciousness, you have the space to defuse your thoughts and feelings and, more importantly, respond to them in a different fashion.

So when we are talking about true Self-consciousness (big S), we are talking about living in a state where you are aware, you understand, and you know yourself as the awareness within. This is not about understanding awareness intellectually. This is much more than a concept in your mind. Instead, you actually live this experience of consciousness firsthand; you observe the mind and body. There is a clear space between you and your mind. You are aware of the mind, the space, and the fact that you are aware. When you are genuinely experiencing awareness-consciousness, it is not something that is done in the mind. It is pure present-moment awareness. You are aware that you are aware.

Dr. Daniel Siegel explained this concept really well in his book called *Aware*:

The mind is like the ocean. And deep in this ocean, beneath the surface, it's calm and clear. And no matter what the surface conditions are, whether flat or choppy or even a full gale storm, deep in the ocean, it's tranquil. From the depth of the ocean, you can look toward the surface and just notice the activity there, as in the mind, where from the depth of the mind you can look upward toward the waves, the brainwaves at the surface of your mind, where all that activity of mind, thoughts, feelings, sensations, and memories exist. You have the incredible opportunity to simply observe those activities at the surface of your mind.

And perhaps my favorite explanation of awareness was presented by Dr. David Hawkins in his book *Letting Go*:

Through inner observation, there is the realization of something that remains constant and the same, no matter what goes on in the external world or with the body, emotions, or mind. With this awareness comes a state of total freedom. The inner Self has been discovered. The silent state of Awareness that underlies all movement, activity, sound, feeling, and thought is discovered to be a timeless dimension of peace. Once identified with this Awareness, we are no longer at the effect of the world, the body, or the mind, and with this Awareness come an inner calmness, stillness, and a profound sense of inner peace. We realize that this is what we were always seeking but didn't know it, because we had gotten lost in the maze. We had mistakenly equated ourselves with the outer phenomena of our hectic life – the body and its experiences, the obligations, the jobs, the titles, the activities, the problems, and the feelings. But now we realize that we are the timeless space in which the phenomena are happening. These progressive realizations of our true nature prepare the ground for the Ultimate Realization of the identity of Consciousness with Divinity Itself.

The Levels of Consciousness

The entire point of all of this is that there are different levels of consciousness that we can experience as human beings. How many in total? I don't know. As of this writing, I am only conscious of the two levels I have discussed. But maybe there are even higher levels of consciousness that I have zero awareness of. But for this book, we will only focus on these two levels.

The lower level would be your small self, or your ego. Living in that level of consciousness means that you are aware, understand, and know yourself as your thoughts, feelings, beliefs, and self-concepts. To draw off the metaphor offered by Dr. Daniel Siegel, you are living on the ocean's surface. This is why people who are ego-conscious use phrases like "I am angry," "I am scared," or "I am depressed." They literally believe themselves to be a feeling. Hopefully, you are beginning to see how untrue a statement like that really is.

The higher level would be your higher self, or awareness-consciousness—being aware of, understanding, and knowing yourself as the awareness within. Drawing again from the ocean metaphor, you are the deep stillness underneath the surface in this scenario.

When you experience a shift into your higher level of consciousness, you become aware, understand, and know yourself as something other than your thoughts and feelings. You are, in fact, the witness, the observer, and the awareness of your thoughts and feelings. You are the one who notices them.

Now, it's necessary to understand that if you are like most people, you can constantly shift between the different levels of consciousness. And you probably will continue to do so for the rest of your life unless you reach enlightenment. But the difference is now you can at least be aware when you shift into a lower level of consciousness. And then you can begin to bring yourself back to your higher self of awareness.

And that, my friend, is the cornerstone of everything I'm writing in this chapter. You are the awareness and observer of your thoughts and feelings. But as the awareness, you can get lost in thoughts and feelings. Getting lost simply means losing your seat of awareness and merging with an object. In the same exact way, you can completely lose yourself in a suspenseful movie or intense game. You can completely forget that you are even watching a show. Pretty wild, huh? This can also happen internally. You can lose your seat of awareness and get lost in your thoughts and feelings.

So if you've been searching for help for a while, bouncing to different programs and books and trying to figure out why you are still stuck, I would like to present the possibility that the tools and methods have not been the primary reason you've struggled on your journey. It is likely because you've been applying them from the wrong level of consciousness. It is so vital that you understand that because you need to be at the level of awareness-consciousness when you apply the Triple-A Response®. Otherwise, it just won't work.

If you're not quite at the stage of conscious awareness yet, one of the best ways to develop this is by practicing being in a state of awareness-consciousness through meditation. We have an awesome meditation series as part of our Taking Back Control Program, and there are tons of meditations all over the internet. The reason I would encourage you to try our program, aside from being heavily biased, is that our meditation program specifically focuses on consciousness and OCD and anxiety.

I want to make one last point relating to shifting in and out of the different levels of consciousness. The more you are in that state of higher consciousness, the easier it is to know when you're in that state of consciousness. Likewise, the more you live in a state of higher consciousness, the easier it is to know when you're not in that state. It really is a practice. It is a different way of going through your life.

So if you practice awareness-consciousness for ten minutes and then go into ego-consciousness for the rest of the day, which one do you think you'll get better at?

By shifting into higher consciousness, we aren't solving OCD and anxiety; we are dissolving it. We are recontextualizing it completely. In fact, we're beginning to understand it as a non-issue. Because if you try to solve OCD from a level of ego-consciousness, from the same level of consciousness from which it was created, you'll have a great deal of difficulty. If you operate from this level of consciousness, you will attempt to use the tools to try to combat the thoughts and feelings. If you do this, you will lose the battle.

Whereas by moving into a higher state of consciousness, you become the observer—you recognize that your response to your thoughts and feelings is separate from you. And when you begin responding to them differently, you won't reinforce the loop. In fact, you'll break the loop altogether and ultimately realize this is not something you need to put any energy into.

With all that said, let's shift into learning and applying the Triple-A Response®. See you in the next chapter.

CHAPTER SEVEN

The Triple-A Response®

"Focus on the solution, not on the problem."

Jim Rohn

Okay, we've talked about a lot of things up to this point. We've discussed the nervous system and psychological stress. We've discussed the OCD & anxiety loop and the lens of fear that develops. We've talked about conditioning, ERP, and neuroplasticity. We've also gone into how safety behaviors keep you stuck in the loop and how we perform most of them mentally. And let's not forget that whole concept of consciousness we covered in the last chapter.

Bottom line, you've gone through a lot of stuff to get to this point, and I hope you can see why that journey was so important. It is the entire foundation on which the Triple-A Response® was developed. Your journey up until now has provided you with the background knowledge to feel confident about why you should implement the Triple-A Response®. So if you just skipped right here, please go back and read the previous chapters. You're only cheating yourself if you don't.

Now let's jump into the real reason you invested in this book.

What Is the Triple-A Response® and How Will It Help You?

Okay, so you understand that OCD and anxiety always (yes, always) work in a loop. And when you get stuck in the loop, you end up engaging in safety behaviors (mental and physical) in an attempt to neutralize intrusive thoughts and anxious feelings. These safety behaviors offer short-term relief but keep you stuck in the loop over the long term. Therefore, the real problem is not the feelings or thoughts but the fact that you are stuck in a loop. And by now we've established the only way to break the loop is by stopping all your safety behaviors, which will break the loop and shift your nervous system back into the parasympathetic (Green) state.

But as you've probably experienced in your life, telling someone to stop unhealthy behaviors, especially behaviors that offer temporary relief, isn't very effective advice. If it was, I would simply tell everyone who wrestles with alcohol dependency to "stop drinking." Problem solved, right?

Same concept with people who are caught in the OCD & anxiety loop. Telling people in the loop to stop doing safety behaviors doesn't work. It is not that easy, and for most humans, that approach simply doesn't work—and the reason is that you still focus your *attention* and *energy* on the problematic behavior. As Tony Robbins—a famous life and business strategist and bestselling author—says, "Where attention goes, energy flows."

That's where the Triple-A Response® comes in. The Triple-A Response® is a solution-focused method that provides a clear path to anchor into and the exact steps to perform every time unwanted thoughts and uncomfortable feelings surface. The critical distinction between what you've been doing and what the Triple-A Response® teaches is that the Triple-A Response® directs you toward what *to* do rather than what *not* to do. And while the difference may sound trivial, I assure you it's not.

Let me explain what I mean. When your intrusive thoughts and feelings pop up, you often **react** and instantly engage in your safety behaviors, usually without even realizing it. The issue with reactivity is that the uncomfortable feeling is the driving force of the behavior. And since you can't always control your thoughts and feelings, this will ultimately lead to you not being in control of your behaviors. If you aren't in control of your behaviors, you're not in control of your life.

You start breaking the loop when you shift to responding rather than reacting. Responding means making a conscious decision rather than reacting with an unconscious impulse. You choose to align your behaviors with your long-term wants and health needs, not respond in a way that only benefits you in the short term (like safety behaviors). And instead of trying not to engage in unhealthy behaviors, you anchor your attention and energy into healthy behaviors that will indirectly prevent harmful behaviors.

From a nervous system perspective, this makes complete sense because when you are in Yellow and your fight-or-flight response is activated, the idea of doing nothing is not really an option. Therefore, the idea of "don't do safety behaviors" doesn't make sense from a purely biological perspective. It leads to people white-knuckling the experience of anxiety, which is still a form of resistance.

On the other hand, when we implement the Triple-A Response®, we are moving in opposition to fear. We are tapping into courage and moving into a solution as opposed to doing nothing. When we are afraid, it helps the mind to have specific steps to anchor into. And by implementing this process, we are sending consistent messages of safety to the brain and nervous system. We are moving to the solution.

To use the alcohol dependency example again, instead of someone telling themself, "I will not drink alcohol," when they go out, it is far better to shift their attention and energy into what *to* do. So maybe when that person goes to a restaurant, they anchor themselves into three simple choices. They are only allowed to order a coffee, a soda water, or an iced tea. By moving into three solutions and only ordering these items, they can never order alcohol. **When they direct their attention and energy toward what *to* do, they move their attention and energy toward a solution rather than operating from a place of resisting a problem.**

The Triple-A Response®: From Problem-Focused to Solution-Focused

Most OCD and anxiety interventions lack a transparent, solution-focused approach. That's precisely why I developed the Triple-A Response®. This method is what I needed when I was stuck and what people who are currently stuck need—a simple, clear solution that focuses on what to do, not what you shouldn't do.

The Triple-A Response® has three straightforward steps:

1. **Agree** and disengage.
2. **Allow** the feelings.
3. **Attack** the fear.

The following three chapters explain each step in detail. My entire road to recovery changed when I switched to a solution-focused approach. I no longer spent my days trying to scrap thoughts, feelings, or even safety behaviors. I just shifted my attention and energy to this solution. And by doing so, I indirectly eliminated the safety behaviors that were spinning the wheel, especially all the mental safety behaviors.

Now, of course there are other interventions and strategies you can use in supplementation with the Triple-A Response®, but this is your main foundation for recovery. In my twelve-week program, Taking Back Control, I incorporate other tools like meditation, somatic experiencing, breathwork, ACT, exposure hierarchies, and mindfulness. Everything has its place and time, but it all builds off the foundation of the Triple-A Response®. Consider the Pareto principle or the 80/20 rule, which states that 80 percent of your results come from 20 percent of the things you do. Some even claim it's more 90/10 or 95/5. Well, the Triple-A Response® is the 20 percent that will produce at least 80 percent of your results, and I would argue more.

It's about working smarter, not harder. You've probably been working very hard to "fix" yourself. By moving to a solution-focused approach, you are switching your thinking to, "What should I do?" rather than, "What should I not do." And when you focus on bringing positivity into your life, you eliminate the negative.

When you follow this approach, your safety behaviors (mental and physical) will be eliminated as a secondary effect. If you practice it consistently, over time, you'll start to notice that your intrusive thoughts and anxious feelings fade as well, but strangely it won't matter as much as you think because your focus will continue to be on controlling the only thing you've ever really had control over . . . your behaviors. This is the effect of applying the Triple-A Response®.

It's a very simple and very effective plan. As Dr. David Hawkins points out in his book *Letting Go*, "Simplicity is the earmark of truth." And the reality is your plan should be simple. Complexity creates confusion. But just because something is simple doesn't mean it's easy to do. It takes concentration, courage, and discipline—all of which you have within you. You are about to transition from a disempowered position to an empowered one—you are about to take back control of your life. So without further ado, let's dive into the first step of the Triple-A Response®: agree and disengage.

Chapter Eight

Step One: Agree and Disengage

"The truth is that there is no actual stress or anxiety in the world; it's your thoughts that create these false beliefs. You can't package stress, touch it, or see it. There are only people engaged in stressful thinking."

Wayne Dyer

When you first read the title of this chapter, you may have thought something to the effect of, "Why on earth would I agree with these thoughts?"

It's the number one question people ask when I present the idea of agreeing and disengaging. It seems foolish even to suggest. To answer this question, we need to discuss the voice inside your head. Let's get started.

The Voice Inside Your Head

Have you noticed that voice inside your head that doesn't shut up? Most of us have a mental dialogue that accompanies us wherever we go. And it doesn't just tell one side of the story, oh no. It often has full-on conversation with itself. This is the voice in our mind.

It plays the role of the devil and the angel, the positive and negative, good and bad. It judges everything. The negative is often louder than the positive—that's what it's like with OCD and anxiety anyway. When the negative is louder, that's typically the one we listen to. This voice is where our what-if and negative intrusive thoughts come from. This is the ego or the small self that we discussed in the chapter on consciousness.

Michael Singer eloquently explains this phenomenon in his book, *The Untethered Soul*. Singer presents the idea of not trying to fight with the voice in your mind and instead learning to watch it and, more importantly, not getting involved. To do this, you need to take a step back from it. This is the concept of shifting into a higher level of consciousness or the higher self. From this seat of awareness, we can begin to see how this voice isn't that great at guiding us through life. In fact, it often produces wildly inaccurate predictions that lead us astray—far away from our core values.

Think about it for a second. With all the worries you've experienced in life, how often has the voice in your head been right? If you're like me, the answer is rarely. So if it's basically never right, then why do we always listen to it as if it is? If we had a financial adviser that was wrong as much as our minds are, would we keep investing our money with them? Hell no, you wouldn't!

So the first step is recognizing that you are not the voice in the mind—you're the one who hears it. Can you remember how you do this? We discussed it in chapter 6. As a reminder, you do this by understanding that the voice is there, and since you hear it, you must be separate from it—you are the one (the awareness) who hears the voice. With this, you shift between the two levels of consciousness: you (the awareness) and the voice you are aware of.

As we discussed in chapter 6, this is what Singer calls the subject-object relationship. You're the subject, and the voice is the object. Because you (the subject) can identify the voice (the object), you are not the same. It is the same way when you look at your coffee mug on your desk. Are you that coffee mug? I assume your answer is no. Your mug is an object you are aware of; it isn't you. It's just an object. You can't be that object. After all, you're aware of it, just like you can't be the voice inside your mind because you are aware of it.

And with this recognition of higher consciousness, you can now change how you respond to the voice in your mind. This is the space where your freedom lies—in this straightforward realization. It's a decision you may not have previously been aware of or even had available to you because you were simply unaware.

But now you are aware, and the instant you become aware, everything changes. Now, you can choose whether or not to engage with the voice of the mind. You can choose whether you metaphorically want to "take the bait."

The Fisherman and the Lure

Several years back, I was learning to fly fish, and my teacher explained how there are different bugs for the fish to eat at different times of the day. To catch a fish, you need to create a lure that looks like the bug that generally lands on the water at the time of day you're fishing. So when you're fly fishing in the morning, you need to craft a lure that looks like the bugs fish eat in the morning, and so on throughout the day.

When you first throw a lure out attempting to catch a fish, you check to see if that lure entices the fish. If you are able to catch a fish with that lure, you're likely to keep catching fish, so you keep using that lure. By that same token, if you throw out a lure and it's not getting any bites over a long period, you may want to consider changing up the lure. If a lure isn't working, the evidence is right there in front of you, so you switch and try a different lure to increase your chances of the fish "taking the bait."

In the context of OCD and anxiety, this is how the voice in the mind works. Our mind is the fisherman, and the intrusive thoughts are like the lures. When we act on them by performing safety behaviors, we're biting and taking the bait. Just like with the fish, biting the lure ultimately leads to us getting caught. So every time you do a safety behavior in response to a particular thought, your mind thinks, "Great, that thought (or lure) worked; let's throw it out again."

Continuing with this analogy, the voice in your mind (the fisherman) throws out lures (what-if thoughts) in an attempt to catch you (the fish). And just like when a real fisherman throws out a lure, the fish has two options—they can bite or just let it be. The fish doesn't have the option of making the lures go away. In the same way, we can't make the intrusive thoughts go away. We only have the option to bite or not to bite.

And what happens when a fisherman catches a fish? They usually get excited, and it motivates them to try to catch more fish, so they throw more lures into the water. What happens when the fisherman doesn't catch a fish? They eventually get bored, give up, and go home. The metaphor here is that if you (the fish) consistently don't bite on the lures (the intrusive thoughts), the fisherman (the mind) gives up and stops throwing out those lures.

This leads us to a very common question . . .

Why do you struggle with your specific theme of intrusive thoughts?

Everyone (and I do mean everyone) I have ever worked with has articulated at some point that they would much rather have a different theme to their OCD and anxiety than the one they deal with. They usually assume that if they did, they could easily implement the tools I teach them. To be honest, I thought the same thing when I was stuck.

This brings us to the question, why do these specific thoughts keep popping into your head? The answer is pretty simple: You (the fish) bit on that lure. You reacted to that particular what-if thought with a safety behavior, which validated it—it made it seem important. In turn, this taught the fisherman (or conditioned the mind) that producing this thought in some way, shape, or form helped keep you safe, which increased the likelihood of your mind using those same what-if thoughts again. The more you have bitten on the lure, the more the fisherman will use it.

At this point, many people ask, "Why does the voice in the mind even exist?" I'm not going to pretend to understand this phenomenon entirely. But my best guess is that at some point in our evolutionary journey, having the ability to predict future threats helped our survival, especially in more primitive times. The problem is, many of us in today's world don't encounter physical threats day in and day out. The voice of the mind attempts to keep us safe, but it can't effectively do so because there are millions of possible threats we may encounter every day.

Additionally, the mind seems to correspond to our nervous system and emotional state. So the more we are in Yellow and Red, the louder the mind seems to get. In his book *Letting Go*, Dr. David Hawkins makes the case that the mind attempts to justify the presence of specific emotional experiences in the body. This is an interesting argument because most people with OCD and anxiety tend to have elevated symptoms during stressful periods of life. I know that was very true of my personal experience.

The overall point is that we must let go of the idea that every thought inside our heads is important. Most of them are utter nonsense—that's the truth. We definitely shouldn't be living our lives, listening to, fighting with, or trying to figure out everything our minds are saying.

But how do we filter out the nonsense? Well . . . we learn to agree and disengage with the mind.

Agree and Disengage: Not Taking the Bait

Let me begin by clearly stating the central message of this step:

When you agree and disengage the thoughts, you do not agree that what your mind is saying is true. Instead, you simply agree and disengage from whatever your intrusive thoughts are saying. You are doing this to avoid getting caught in the conversation. You are doing this from a place of awareness-consciousness.

In this stage of the Triple-A Response®, we're getting those what-if thoughts that the mind comes up with, then just agreeing and disengaging from them. The aim of this is to shut down the conversation completely by becoming disinterested. We just stop engaging with the what-if thoughts altogether. It's not to say, "Ah, yes, I agree with what you're saying; I will act immediately." That's the total opposite of what I mean.

Let me offer an analogy that will help clear any confusion here.

Imagine you have an overly political relative. You don't have to see them very often, but when you do, you just try to get through without making it weird. You know their political views are different from yours, and you're aware there's no point discussing politics with them because it never ends well. You decide to outfox them and avoid conflict—you just agree and disengage with whatever they say. The reason is that for an argument to exist, there must be two opposing sides. When you agree and disengage, you stop the conversation before it ever begins, to shut them up. You choose to take the high road.

Have you ever been trying to share something with someone and they just looked completely disinterested in what you are saying?

You know how deflating that feels?

That's exactly what we are doing with the mind.

But for this work, you have to be consistent. You have to stay the course and not engage even when they say things you don't agree with. Even when they try to coax you in with a particularly controversial statement, you just agree and disengage, agree and disengage. Always remember it takes two to tango. An argument can only exist if there are two sides. If you refuse to provide the second side, the conflict can't happen.

In this scenario and any other where you agree and disengage, you are in no way demonstrating that you agree with the content of the conversation. You are still able to retain your actual beliefs and points of view. You are just refusing to engage—that's the entire point of this step.

When it comes to OCD and anxiety, this is not about letting your OCD and anxiety win. It's not telling the voice in your mind that you agree with what the intrusive thoughts are saying. You're just pacifying them by deciding not to engage in a conversation. You are metaphorically not taking the bait that the fisherman is throwing.

So let's say you touch a doorknob, and the voice in your mind says, "What if I get XYZ disease?" When you implement this first step, you might say something to the effect of, "Yeah, OK, whatever," and move on because you know this isn't a disease issue; it's an OCD & anxiety loop issue.

By agreeing and disengaging, you don't get into this constant back-and-forth of whether you're going to get sick or not or how to prevent getting sick; you do none of that. You don't give your what-if thoughts any airtime—you accept getting sick as one possibility of a billion different things that could happen in life, and there are also a million different variables that are all beyond your control, and you move on.

Again, let me stress that you don't have to agree with or like the things the mind is saying. That's not the point. You just have to briefly notice whatever the mind says and refuse to do anything about it. Because the thing is, when we get into an argument with the mind, we are already engaged in our mental safety behaviors. The moment we get into the conversation, our higher awareness gets lost in the ego. We can no longer separate ourselves from the voice. That's what I mean when I talk about getting lost in the loop. You, the awareness, lose your seat of awareness and get lost in the conversation of the mind.

When you refuse to engage, you are responding instead of reacting. You recognize that the problem is much bigger than what the what-if thought is saying, even if it's a bunch of the same what-if thoughts repeatedly! You acknowledge that your thoughts and feelings aren't the problems. The problem is the loop. And the loop forms because of all the safety behaviors you do in response to these thoughts and feelings, especially all those mental safety behaviors like rumination, mental review, analyzing, thought blocking, thought suppression, and so on.

The only way to move toward the solution and not away from the problem is to not get into the discussion at all. When I started doing this, it felt like my what-if thoughts were never-ending, like they would keep popping up forever. I had to continually remind myself why I was doing what I was doing. If I got involved, I would end up lost in that loop and the world of OCD and anxiety. And I knew that was not a place I wanted to be.

So however hard it might feel to agree and disengage, it is absolutely a choice you have. Just remind yourself not to take the bait. The voice in your mind is trying to lure you in and get you to bite. That's what it does. You cannot stop the mind. But you do have the choice not to take the bait. Just let it be there in front of you and don't bite. Trust me, the more you do this, the easier it gets. Practice makes progress.

It's going to seem counterintuitive at first. It did for me too. Do not try to outthink this. Do not let the mind tell you that it can't be this simple. I know it seems too simple, and that's the entire point. I know your mind will say, "Yeah, but what about these XYZ important thoughts? What do I do with those?" Agree and disengage them. That's just a lure trying to convince you there are specific intrusive thoughts that are important.

The reality is that once your mind calms down and you feel more like yourself again, you can revisit whatever you are worried about and determine if you want to address it then from a higher level of consciousness. But in my experience, you will likely see it as a non-issue because the lens of fear will have lifted. Then you can look at whatever you are worried about from a clear place and respond with your pure intuition.

For now, the goal is to stay out of the conversation altogether. And just to prepare you, this first step brings a lot of fear and anxiety to the surface, which can feel overwhelming. But don't worry! That's what step number two, *allow the feelings*, is all about. So meet me in the next chapter so we can dive into it.

CHAPTER NINE

Step Two: Allowing the Anxiety

"I must not fear. Fear is the mind-killer. Fear is the little-death that brings total obliteration. I will face my fear. I will permit it to pass over me and through me. And when it has gone past I will turn the inner eye to see its path. Where the fear has gone there will be nothing. Only I will remain."

Frank Herbert, Dune

Your body is insanely smart, and it knows how to heal itself. In fact, that is what it is doing twenty-four hours a day, even while you sleep. It knows how to breathe without you thinking about it. It knows how to circulate your blood and repair injuries without you thinking about it. It knows how to take the food you eat, turn it into fuel for your body, and expel the waste afterward. It does this, all without you ever consciously thinking about it. And guess what? In this same way, it knows what to do when you experience different emotions in your body.

Why does this matter? Well, the fundamental cornerstone of this second step in the Triple-A Response® is to trust your body and its ability to process emotions—to allow it to experience and release the energy, whatever that energy may be. In the case of

OCD and anxiety, it's primarily about having trust that your body knows what to do with all the fear and anxiety you are experiencing, without you attempting to control it.

Sometimes when I start talking about energy, I get a lot of eye rolls and sideways glances. Maybe even a comment, like, "Oh great, some energy freak again," like I've somehow crossed a barrier from the real world to the imaginary fantasy land of energy healing.

For some reason (I have my suspicions that Big Pharma is somehow involved), the West collectively likes to downplay or ignore the role of energy when it comes to health. But the reality is everything is energy. In fact, the very first law of thermodynamics is that energy cannot be created or terminated, merely transmitted from one thing to the next (Zohuri, 2018). Now, we *could* dive deeper into the field of quantum physics and explore energy from the level of protons and neutrons if we wanted to. But don't worry, we won't.

Instead, let's use some good old critical thinking. First, think about how your heart beats all day long, your blood circulates through your body, your body processes food, and all your organs work diligently to help your body function. This happens day in and day out without you giving it a second thought. All of these processes require energy. Have you ever asked yourself where that energy comes from? Or what is the source of that energy that is keeping you alive? As I stated above, according to the first law of thermodynamics, your body doesn't create the energy, it receives and transmits energy.

Further, when people undergo PET scans, the scan measures energy levels in different brain regions. So you are constantly experiencing energy coursing through your body. Still, for some reason, the mention of energy and health together sends people running for the hills.

The point I'm making is, energy is real, energy is undeniable, energy is everything. Now, what does energy have to do with emotion and our body? Well, let's do a quick history lesson. The word *emotion* dates back to the 1100s and is derived from the French word *émouvoir*, which, when translated, means "to stir up." To stir up what? Well, the only answer I can think of is energy.

Then, in the 1800s, Thomas Brown coined the word *emotion*. This means emotions weren't even part of our working language until about two hundred years ago. Isn't that kind of wild? Before we started talking about emotion, people would use phrases to describe certain behaviors, like "acts of passion."

So what is an emotion? The current Lexico definition of *emotion* is "a strong feeling deriving from one's circumstances, mood, or relationships with others." That's a pretty good starting place, but even in that definition, "a strong feeling" is kind of presented as a thing or used as a noun. But the thing is, you can't see, hear, or touch a feeling, and feelings are generally experienced totally differently by two separate individuals. For instance, if you said you were feeling anxious, and I said I was feeling nervous, are we really feeling the exact same way? Probably not.

Feelings are hard to define and discuss within our language— and especially back then! During the 1970s, psychologist Paul Ekman identified six basic emotions: happiness, sadness, disgust, fear, surprise, and anger (Ekman, 1999). In 2015, Pixar made a great movie on these basic emotions called *Inside Out*, although they left out surprise in the movie. And while there is still a general agreement that we only have a few basic emotions, we also understand that each of these feelings can expand on an entire continuum.

In fact, psychotherapist Michael C. Graham advocates that all emotions exist on a continuum of intensity (Wikipedia, 2022). Therefore, fear might range from mild concern to absolute terror, whereas shame might range from simple embarrassment to toxic shame. This is exactly why I discussed the spectrum of psychological stress in chapter 3 and made an argument for letting go of all these different anxiety disorders.

The point is that feelings are often difficult to discuss and process because they are challenging to define and communicate—we don't have sufficient language to articulate them. They exist in the body, not in the mind. But it is imperative that we, as humans, can process and metabolize emotions in our bodies in a healthy way, or it will create dis-ease. There is sufficient research to suggest that the physical diseases we experience in the body strongly correlate to emotional dis-ease that we have stored in the mind (Mental Health Foundation, 2022).

If you are interested in going deeper on the topic of emotional dis-ease and its connection to physical disease, two of my recommended books to start with would be *When the Body Says No* by Gabor Maté, and *Dying to Be Me* by Anita Moorjani.

Instead of trying to come up with perfect definitions for this book and the application of the Triple-A Response®, I want you to let go of spending your time trying to label your emotions. Instead, I want you to switch to calling emotions, *energy*. Remember it like this, *e-motion* is just energy-in-motion in your body. It is the actual sensations you are experiencing in this moment.

I want you to do this for two reasons. One, feelings are meant to be felt in the body, not thought about in the mind. In the book

Letting Go, Dr. David Hawkins explains how most of the time, when you try to identify and process feelings in the thinking mind, it draws you away from experiencing the feeling in your body. He explains in the book that letting go of emotions is actually about bringing your full awareness into the feelings. I think one of the primary reasons people have trouble feeling their feelings is that they actually avoid them by trying to think and talk about them.

Two, energy is neutral. It just is. Energy is not good or bad. Energy exists in specific vibrational patterns and frequencies. We might experience some energy in a low vibration, and some might be in a high vibration, but both forms of energy are not good or bad; they just are. You already know this. Think about it. When you say you like someone's vibe, what are you actually saying? You like the energetic vibration they are transmitting and you are receiving. In most cases, no words even need to be said for you to pick up the energy of another person.

One of the main reasons people resist their feelings so much is because they maintain false beliefs about the existence of different "good' and "bad' feelings. Most people think they are only supposed to feel "good." And if they don't feel "good," then that is "bad," and therefore, if they feel a "bad feeling," they need to get rid of the "bad feeling" so they can feel good. But this begs the following two questions: Is there such a thing as a "bad feeling?" And if there are "bad feelings," who said that feeling these "bad feelings" are actually "bad?"

MATT'S TINFOIL HAT MOMENT

There are only two countries in the *entire* world where pharmaceutical companies can legally advertise prescription-level drugs directly to public consumers. Those two countries are the United States and New Zealand. Now, I am wearing my tin foil hat writing this.

Under this hat, I had this crazy thought that maybe these companies stood to profit somehow and benefit from convincing a large number of people that a normal energetic experience was abnormal. Oh wait, never mind. That's crazy; we've never seen any evidence where pharmaceutical companies would prioritize profit over the health and safety of the individual person. Just kidding, of course we have! Don't you dare look up things like the Tuskegee Experiment. That's it! I'm done wearing this hat—I need to fall back in line. After all, I don't want weird men in black suits showing up at my house and taking me away.

Anyway, back to the book.

The best way, I believe, to challenge the ideas that some feelings are good and others bad is to stop labeling our feelings and simply call them energy.

The energy in your body changes constantly. It may be high; it may be low, but it really doesn't matter. Your job is simply to be with whatever energy you are experiencing and let it go.

Discharging (Stress) Energy

No one knows about stress quite like neurobiologist Dr. Robert Sapolsky. In his book, *Why Zebras Don't Get Ulcers*, he gives perhaps one of the most comprehensive breakdowns of stress and its impact on the body. As we discussed earlier in the book, stress is simply our body's response to a challenge or threat (real or perceived)—the *fight-or-flight response*. In his book, Dr. Sapolsky discusses how our stress response essentially puts our normal bodily function in reverse or upside down.

Simply put, when the stress response is activated (Yellow), our body needs as much energy as possible. Our bodies take all the energy in our bloodstream and direct it into specific functions (like our large muscle groups) to help us survive in that moment. That makes sense, right? If you're in danger, your body needs to focus on running or fighting, not reproducing or healing. This massive energy spike enables us to spring into action, either by fighting or running away.

So how do zebras fit in? Well, unfortunately for zebras, there are all sorts of other animals that like to eat them for dinner. Since zebras have a lot of predators, they spend a lot of time in the stress response. When a zebra senses a threat, such as a lion near them, their body activates the stress response and propels them to get out of Dodge.

As they run away, they're either mowed down and eaten by the lion, or they outrun the lion and reach a place of safety. At this point, their bloodstream is full of energy because that's what is necessary to flee the lion. But if kept in the body for a long time afterward, the stress energy can be harmful. Therefore, if the zebra reaches a safe space, their body needs to find a way to return to its normal state, also known as *homeostasis*.

A zebra intuitively understands that it can't keep all that energy in the body, as it'll cause many unhealthy side effects, like ulcers (hence the title of Dr. Sapolsky's book.) So what does the zebra do? It shakes off and discharges the energy to release the stress from its body. Once the stress energy is entirely gone, the zebra often, almost instantly, snaps back to grazing like nothing ever happened.

This isn't uncommon in the animal world. You've probably seen a dog shake before. Dr. Peter Levine explains how deer do this in his book, *Walking the Tiger: Healing Trauma*. He describes what he saw when observing the deer—it starts with twitching their necks, then their chests, right down to their hind legs. This muscle vibration regulates the body, switching off the sympathetic nervous system and returning to a relaxed state, where the parasympathetic nervous system takes over.

Physically shaking themselves free from stress is how these mammals sidestep the long-term effects of stress. They feel the stress, release it, and return to a calm state. Children tend to naturally do this when they are afraid. But unfortunately, it seems that somewhere between childhood and adulthood, many humans forget to do this. Instead of releasing the stress when it surfaces, we engage in behaviors that either perpetuate it or suppress it in our bodies.

But rest assured, you can release stress energy from your body. I will not pretend to understand exactly how this energetic process works, but I know from personal experience that there are times when I have had vast surges of anxious energy in my body. And I also know that I am no longer experiencing that particular energetic vibration, which means at some point between the onset of the feeling and now, that energy must have left my body.

Where did that energy go? I don't know, and to be transparent, I don't really care. I have never lost a wink of sleep over this question, and you shouldn't either. Remember the first law of thermodynamics: Energy can't be created, merely transferred. That's all that happens when you allow emotions (energy in motion) to surface in your body. When you become fully aware of a feeling in your body, think of it as a gateway where you have the opportunity to transfer the energy out of your body.

Fight or Flight (or Freeze)?

I'm not going to spend a lot of time on this concept, but I felt it essential to at least mention it while we are on this subject. In his fascinating book, which I referenced above, *Waking the Tiger: Healing Trauma*, Dr. Peter Levine discusses how this bodily processing of stress heals trauma. Specifically, the technique of somatic experiencing. In the book, Dr. Levine explicitly discusses the stress response's highest level: the freeze response (Red). The freeze response is activated when our bodies determine that neither fighting nor fleeing will keep us safe. It is our last-ditch effort for survival.

The main thing to know about the freeze response is it is directly linked to the experience of trauma. When a person enters the freeze response (Red), internally, their body is still reacting to the threatening situation like it would if they were to fight or flee. It makes all that energy readily available to fight or flee. The difference is, when you freeze, you don't utilize it. This causes the excess energy to get stuck and stored in the body, ultimately leading to trauma.

This process is relevant if you are experiencing symptoms of trauma or post-traumatic stress disorder. If that is the case, it's nothing to get overwhelmed about. It means you should consider adding techniques specifically related to trauma and the body, like *somatic experiencing* or *trauma-releasing exercises* (TRE), to your recovery practice. I discuss this more in-depth in my Taking Back Control Program.

But for the vast majority of people reading this book, the primary focus of your work is really going to be about learning to simply allow your feelings to surface in your body. With that said, let's move into the second step of the Triple-A Response®—allowing the anxiety.

Step Two: Allowing the Anxiety

So just like in step one, let me begin by clearly stating the central message of this step of the Triple-A Response®:

When you allow feelings in your body, you are *not* allowing the feeling to make it go away. Instead, you are bringing your awareness into your body and your awareness into the actual feelings and sensations in your body. Then you are giving the feeling permission to come to the surface. Then, when it does, you experience the feeling in its entirety. And just like in step one, you are doing this from a place of awareness-consciousness.

When explaining this concept to my clients, I like to refer back to *Harry Potter and the Sorcerer's Stone*. In the book and movie, Harry, Ron, and Hermione are searching for the Sorcerer's Stone. After they get through the trap door guarded by the three-headed dog, they get stuck in this large group of vines called Devil's Snare.

Now Devil's Snare is tricky because as Harry and Ron start to resist and try to get out of the Devil's Snare, the plant begins to constrict, binding their arms and legs. In other words, the more they resist and fight being stuck, the more stuck they become. Luckily, Hermione comes to the rescue, telling Harry and Ron to relax. She says that if they do, the Devil's Snare will loosen its hold on them, allowing them to get free. Hermione demonstrates this and easily breaks out, and then Harry does the same. Unfortunately for Ron, he can't calm himself down, so Hermione has to come to his aid with a spell.

This is an excellent analogy for anxiety because most of us resist anxiety when it surfaces. We fight against it and clinch up, just like Ron, trying to rid ourselves of it. But paradoxically, that keeps us stuck, just like Devil's Snare. We fight and fight and end up worse off than at the beginning.

Here's the problem: We're not trusting our bodies and as a result, we prevent a natural process from occurring. By allowing your body to feel anxiety naturally, you're permitting your body to let it go. Now, yes, this is uncomfortable initially, but it's a short-term discomfort.

Remember, anxiety (or energy) is normal. It is just a thing that you are experiencing. You'll only strengthen the wheel if you try to get rid of it. By learning to trust your body to experience and release the anxiety on its own accord, you're allowing energy to hit the surface and be released.

How Do I Allow Anxiety?

The question that usually comes up at this point is, "How do I allow anxiety?" Well, first, I want you to notice how you immediately shifted to thinking about allowing your feelings instead of feeling them in your body. Remember, emotions are meant to be felt in the body, not thought about in the mind. You can't feel feelings in your mind. Second, the problem with this question is, it is phrased incorrectly.

It presents *allow* as a verb or an action you would take. The question, "How do I allow anxiety?" implies you need to do something to properly allow your feelings. But in fact, all you need to do is sit back and let the natural motion of energy unfold. You don't need to do anything—it requires no specific action from your end.

The truth is, allowing is not an action; if anything, allowing is inaction. Think about it: What do you have to do in order to allow me to wear the white T-shirt I am currently wearing? Nothing.

What do you have to do to allow a group of people to protest? Nada. What do you have to do to allow the waves to crash on the beach? Nothing. So what do you have to do to allow feelings in your body? Nothing. When you allow something, you consciously decide not to resist or attempt to change it in any way.

Think about allowing a friend to stay at your house for a while. What do you really have to do to make that happen? The reality is you don't have to do anything. They'll ask if they can stay, you'll say, "Sure," and that's it. If you allow them to stay, you won't wander around asking, "Are you still here?" or, "When are you going to leave?" You will just let them be as they are, and they will leave whenever they are ready.

So when I say, "Allow the anxiety," I'm really saying, feel the feeling and let it be there. Do not resist it or try to change it in any way. I'll say this again to stress the importance: Feelings are meant to be felt in your body. That is how the nervous system metabolizes a feeling. Emotions are not meant to be thought about in your head. Upon practicing this more and more, you will realize that feelings are not dangerous—they are just energy. And your body knows what to do. You just need to get out of the way.

No doubt, you have been trying to get rid of and control your feelings for a long time. But I'm telling you, you don't need to do that anymore. Just feel the anxiety; remind yourself it is just energy. It is not dangerous—it just is. It is not good or bad. By all means, you can be aware of its presence, but when it comes to action, choose inaction—allow it to do whatever it needs to do.

When you feel your feelings and allow them to be present, you're teaching your brain that the feelings, and the thoughts that preceded them, aren't dangerous. Over time, your brain will adapt to this through the phenomenon of neuroplasticity, and it'll recognize that it was a false alarm. I know this might sound scary at first, but the more you practice allowing the energy in your body to surface and pass, the easier it will get. Eventually, you'll wonder why you ever tried to control it in the first place.

It will take practice, but you will get there with time. If I can do it and other people before you can do it, you can too!

Once you've begun to truly allow your feelings, it is time to move to our third and final step: Attacking the anxiety. Are you ready?

Meet me over in the next chapter.

CHAPTER TEN

Step Three: Attacking the Anxiety

"Bran thought about it. 'Can a man still be brave if he's afraid?'"
"That is the only time a man can be brave,' his father told him."

George R. R. Martin, A Game of Thrones

To start this chapter, let's go back to the quote by Franklin D. Roosevelt that I mentioned in chapter 2, "The only thing we have to fear is fear itself."

I believe President Roosevelt understood that when we lose ourselves in fear, we aren't in control of our lives. Fear is in control. Fear is the one steering your ship, and as a result, you are a metaphorical passenger along for the ride in your life. I know that sounds harsh, but be honest with yourself for a minute. When you lose yourself in fear, your sole purpose becomes to mitigate an internal feeling state rather than live the way you wish to. You completely lose yourself. This is precisely why the things or situations we are afraid of pale in comparison to the imprisonment of being stuck in a state of fear of that thing or situation.

It's important to remember that anyone can get lost in fear at any point in their life. It's something you can bounce in and out of. In fact, in 2020, we got front-row seats to see the largest display of what happens when the masses get lost in fear. Try to think back to some completely irrational behavior you saw or even personally engaged in during that time period. If you are honest, I think you will agree that it is pretty frightening to witness how the grips of fear can really take over.

Now, I am in no way saying this with any judgment. I've been pretty transparent that I, too, lived many years of my life in fear. There was a time when fear was the primary driving force of my life. I probably wouldn't have admitted it back then, but it was true nonetheless. I just wasn't aware of it. I truly thought I was being logical when I spent all those days engaging in safety behaviors from morning 'til night.

Then, there was a pivotal moment on my road to recovery. That moment came when I had the following realization:

Living in chronic fear of something is actually far worse than the thing itself happening.

Paulo Coelho, in his book *The Alchemist*, said it better when he wrote, "Tell your heart that the fear of suffering is worse than the suffering itself. And that no heart has ever suffered when it goes in search of its dreams, because every second of the search is a second's encounter with God and with eternity."

I finally understood what Roosevelt was saying almost ninety years ago. Fear is the thing we need to fear. Because when we lose ourselves in fear, we lose ourselves completely. Upon this realization, I recognized that it wouldn't be enough to just agree and disengage the mind and allow my anxiety. I had to take an actual stand and move in opposition to my fear. I had to fight back. I had to fight for control of my life.

This is why the third and final step of the Triple-A Response® is to attack the fear. To attack, you have to shift internally from a timid (fearful) stance to a courageous one. And this means inviting the thoughts and feelings you've been most afraid of having come to the surface and making the courageous decision to face them head-on whenever they show up. Then and only then you will truly begin taking back control of your life.

You may think this sounds a little crazy. In fact, you might even feel compelled to stop the book and move on to another program or book. That's OK—notice that resistance—that's the fear I am speaking of, right there. You see, by voluntarily confronting your fear, you are the one initiating the battle. You are cutting the head off the snake. You are becoming the aggressor who's punching in the fight, not the one receiving the blows. And the most crucial thing attacking does? It forces you to drop all your resistance to OCD and anxiety and face it head-on in its entirety.

Speaking of cutting the head off a snake, let's use the fear of snakes as an example. Let's pretend that I was absolutely terrified of snakes. Now, imagine four big men grabbed me and threw me into a room where there was a real, live, poisonous snake on the ground slithering around. How do you think I would respond in that situation? Probably not very well, right? I'd probably be full of resistance and fear. The fear might even be so overwhelming that I become paralyzed (or, in other words, enter into the freeze or Red response).

Now let's visualize a different scenario. Let's pretend I have decided I am sick of my fear of snakes controlling me and want to face it. I voluntarily walk into a room where a poisonous snake is slithering around on the floor and close the door behind me.

In both scenarios, I wind up in the same situation: I am in a confined room with a snake on the ground. In both scenarios, I will likely experience a significant surge of fear in my body. But how I respond to that fear will be very different. This is because in the second scenario, I am tapping into courage and deciding to confront the fear on my terms. Therefore, the fear can't catch me off guard. In essence, I am dropping my resistance to fear. I am deciding not to let fear control me. No one else is choosing this for me, as only I can make this decision. In the same way, no one can make you face your fear. You are the only one who can truly do it.

The big difference between the two scenarios is the choice to engage fear willingly. By choosing the confrontation, I am choosing to face fear itself head-on. And that choice is everything on this journey to recovery.

When facing intrusive thoughts and anxious feelings, you don't have a choice on whether or not you will confront them, but you do get to choose *how* you confront them. You can either face them on your terms or their terms. That is the only real choice you have in the matter.

From Victim to Victor

I am a big fan of retired Navy SEAL commander Jocko Willink. I've learned a lot from his books and his podcast, The Jocko Podcast. On the show, Jocko Willink invites guests on and explores different topics related to war, jujitsu, and personal development. In episode 112, Jocko interviews Dr. Jordan Peterson. They discuss the idea of facing your fears.

I am paraphrasing a part of the episode here—it's not word for word. For the full experience, check it out for yourself. (There's a link in the reference section). In the episode, Dr. Jordan Peterson explains how your nervous system responds entirely differently when you voluntarily face life's demands rather than involuntarily face them. In other words, your internal state matters when confronting a challenge. When you come face-to-face with a challenge, you have the choice to respond to it head-on, or brace yourself for whatever the challenge may do to you and hope for the best. As you can imagine, taking the latter stance will lead to a very disempowered state.

In the episode, Jocko elaborates on this idea as he discusses his experience during his past military deployments. Jocko explains the differences he noticed in the mindset of soldiers on an assault-oriented mission, in contrast to soldiers on patrol or defensive missions. He explained how on assault missions, he saw that soldiers viewed themselves as the threat—they were the ones who were going to inflict damage, kill, and destroy the enemy. Therefore, they were the ones who their opponents should fear.

Conversely, when the soldiers were on patrol or defensive missions, they viewed the enemy as the threat and themselves as waiting for the attack. Therefore, the enemy was the one who they should fear. This mentality put the soldiers in an entirely different internal state.

Now, I want to be very clear here: I am addressing all the men and women who served in the military directly here, especially those who have been deployed and engaged in the horrors of war. I am in no way comparing the experience of actual war with battling OCD and anxiety.

> I am simply drawing from the examples within Jocko's interview and identifying some loose similarities that I feel apply to engaging with fear from a general perspective.

The example above is, I believe, a perfect example of what it means to face fear at the highest level possible.

The point I am making is that we often take a defensive and resistant stance when facing intrusive thoughts, anxious feelings, and triggering situations. By doing this, we get hammered continually by an onslaught of intrusive thoughts and anxious feelings. But when we transition to an offensive stance, we enter the conflict willingly. We eliminate the resistance of the conflict itself and ultimately experience a much better outcome.

I am sure you know this by now, but trying to avoid conflict with OCD and anxiety doesn't work. After all, if it did, you probably wouldn't be reading this book. The choice you have isn't *if* you're going to deal with it. It's simply *how*. You get to decide which side of the conflict you will be on. Are you going to be the victim or the victor? Are you going to play defense or offense? The choice is yours.

Step Three: Attack the Anxiety

So just like in steps one and two, let me begin by clearly stating the central message of step three: Attack the anxiety.

When attacking anxiety, you move directly toward your intrusive thoughts and anxious feelings. This step's key point is that it comes down to your internal intention. You must attack wholeheartedly. It requires courage and total commitment to move against your resistance to your fear. By doing so, you are dropping all opposition and confronting your fear head-on. And just as in steps one and two, you are doing this from a place of awareness-consciousness.

How Do You Attack the Anxiety?

Chances are, right now, you might be feeling resistance. Most people are totally fine with steps 1 and 2, but they get introduced to step 3 (Attack) and want nothing to do with it. However, seeing as you made it this far, I want to ask you to take a little leap of faith, trust me, and continue reading.

Okay, so how do you attack your anxiety?

In my experience, there are several ways to do this. The correct method for you will depend on your specific fears. That said, I am going to introduce three of my favorite strategies when it comes to attacking anxiety:

1. Invite your symptoms to get worse.
2. Take your fears to a scarier place.
3. Purposely move in opposition to your fear.

Okay, let's dive in.

Inviting OCD and Anxiety to Get Worse

Albert Einstein famously stated, "Insanity is doing the same thing repeatedly and expecting different results." If you've been doing safety behaviors for any length of time, this quote should resonate with you. Trying to manage our OCD and anxiety with safety behaviors doesn't work. So the question is, why do we keep doing them? What change are we expecting to experience?

The reality is that you can keep doing safety behaviors and hope for a different outcome, or you can shift your strategy and take an offensive stance. When you invite the OCD and anxiety to get worse, you are taking an internal "bring it on" approach, so to speak. That's what I mean by inviting OCD and anxiety to get worse.

If intrusive thoughts pop up, you invite them to stay as long as they want. Even better, you encourage your brain to produce more of them. And if your anxious feelings are ramping up, you invite the energy to course through your body.

Or, even better than all that, you invite the sensations to intensify. If you start having physical sensations, you also encourage those to intensify. If you notice yourself starting to sweat, you invite your body to sweat even more.

Hopefully you get the point. Again, just like everything else in this book, keep it simple for yourself. Don't overthink this. Your brain is going to want to try to complicate this. Don't let it.

The central point is to drop all your resistance to your present experience—to move with whatever is happening internally. By doing this, you refuse to run away from your experience, and instead, you move right toward it.

When you resist intrusive thoughts and anxious feelings, they weigh you down even more. However, when you face them head-on, you become more courageous, and as you grow, your OCD and anxiety have less power over you.

So that's the first option. The second option is taking the thoughts to a scarier place.

Taking Your Fears to a Scarier Place

If the last section sounded strange, then this concept likely stirs up even more feelings of doubt. But remember, everything on this journey is a complete paradox.

To explain this idea, I will draw from the book *OCD Treatment Through Storytelling* by Dr. Alan Weg. In this book, Dr. Weg draws from a scene in the popular movie *8 Mile*, starring Eminem. So this example is pretty meta, as I am referencing a movie, described in a book, in my own book, but I want to make sure I give credit where credit is due.

At the end of the movie *8 Mile*, Eminem enters a rap battle with the reigning champion, Papa Doc. In case you've never been in a rap battle (like me), rap battles are when two rap artists go head-to-head and insult each other in front of a crowd. The aim of the rap battle is to insult your opponent better than they insult you in your rap.

Anyways, in the movie, Eminem ends up going first, and he proceeds to do the unthinkable. He completely goes off course— instead of insulting Papa Doc, he primarily targets himself. Eminem spends almost his entire time making fun of himself in front of the crowd and Papa Doc. Then once it's Papa Doc's turn, he has nothing to say because everything he was going to say, Eminem already said. He drops the microphone without saying a word, and Eminem wins by default.

This is the approach we take when we take our fears to a scarier place. By willingly taking your fear to an even worse scenario in your mind, you're taking the ammunition OCD and anxiety have in their back pocket and using it on yourself.

To use another example, let's say someone was bullying me in school and told me my shirt was ugly. Instead of defending my shirt, I might try this strategy and tell him, "Yeah, my shirt's ugly, and you know what? My face is ugly, too, and no girl will ever like me, let alone marry me, so I'll probably be alone forever."

Now, do I believe that? No, of course not. But when I take it to a crazy level like that right away, what else can the bully say? You see, by making it worse on purpose, I'm not only stopping the conversation but also challenging the bully. So apply this to your fear—instead of surrendering to it, simply make it worse on purpose and beat the doubt bully to the punch.

This strategy may not be for you and is not always applicable to everyone, but it can be very effective. Again, do not overthink this—don't let your mind complicate it. Now let's move on to the third option.

Actively Defying OCD and Anxiety

The last option I want to discuss is the act of explicitly defying what your fear says. We move in a deliberate, defiant way and literally do the opposite of what our anxious thoughts are telling us to do. This is the ultimate stage of the attack.

One of the funny things about OCD and anxiety is they always tell you how to get better, indirectly, by telling you what not to do. OCD and anxiety actually always show you the way to get better by shining a light on the wrong path. The good news is it is very consistent. This means you can figure out the correct path because it's the opposite of what your fear is saying.

Think about it: Your fear always directs you to engage in a safety behavior, right? And since your goal is to eliminate all safety behaviors, if you do the opposite of what your fear says, you can never engage in a safety behavior. You just have to flip everything on its head. Instead of doing what your fearful thoughts tell you, you do the opposite. It really is that simple.

For example, if your anxiety tells you to avoid social situations, go and stand smack bang in the middle of a crowd or go to the party that scares you. You do this for the simple act of defying your fear, not to make yourself feel better. By doing this, you're saying, "I'm not doing my safety behaviors, and I'm no longer falling victim to my fears."

Again, don't overthink this.

The only way you can ever be sure you're not reinforcing the loop is by moving in opposition to what your fear is telling you to do. If you're terrified of touching a doorknob, put your hand on that doorknob. If you are afraid of speaking in front of people, purposely find ways to practice it.

Now, let's be clear here: This is not easy or comfortable. However, this approach is incredibly effective because you actively face fear head-on at every opportunity you get. That's the only way to break that loop for good. Attacking is the only logical option. Otherwise, we'll continue to get attacked.

Choose to be the victor, not the victim. By doing that, you take an empowered stance over your fear. Trust me, you'll become braver for it. This is not about eliminating your thoughts, because we know that's impossible. This is not about getting rid of your anxious feelings either. Both of those only feed into the wheel.

This is about ensuring you stop *all* of your safety behaviors. If you eliminate all your safety behaviors, the OCD-and-anxiety wheel can't spin. If the wheel stops spinning, you shift your body into the parasympathetic nervous system. Once you do that, the lens of fear lifts. And once the lens of fear lifts, you finally see with clarity that it wasn't what you were afraid of that was the problem, but the fear itself. By breaking free from the grips of fear, you take back control of your life.

The absolute best way to eliminate *all* of your safety behaviors is to start applying a solution-focused approach, the Triple-A Response®.

Agreeing with uncertainty, allowing your anxious thoughts, and attacking your anxiety will ensure you aren't engaging in any mental or physical safety behaviors. And ultimately, this will free you up to take back control of your life and pursue the things that matter to you.

Now, if you find yourself having questions or concerns, that is totally normal. I'd be surprised if you didn't. That's why this is not a journey you should walk alone. It is important to have guidance at all stages of your life. We're not meant to walk through life alone, especially in challenging times. For this reason, the next chapter is full of potential next steps for you. See you there!

What To Do Next?

Well, my friend, we've reached the end of this stage of our journey together. I sincerely hope that you've benefited (and continue to benefit!) from this book.

Let's recap what we've covered:

1. In **Chapter 1**, we took a deep dive into my personal experience with the OCD & anxiety loop. My goal was to show you my lived experience. Therefore, what I cover in this book isn't just some theory—I developed this process out of necessity and out of real-life experience. I have been in the loop. I know how terrifying it can be. But because of this experience, I also know that you can break free.

2. In **Chapter 2**, we talked about the four components that form the OCD & anxiety loop and all the different ways that the loop can manifest. It is so vital that you understand the loop and see the loop as your problem, not the content of your fear.

3. In **Chapter 3**, we talked about the nervous system and your internal stoplight. We also talked about when the OCD & anxiety loop spins, the lens of fear develops and takes over. We went through what it is like to get stuck in that lens of fear and how it distorts your entire world.

4. In **Chapter 4**, we discussed three major shifts you need to make to change how you understand the OCD & anxiety loop, and the importance of seeing this as a behavior problem, as it helps you to focus your energy and attention on things in your control.

5. In **Chapter 5**, we uncovered all the different ways that safety behaviors can show up in your life and, more specifically, the various mental safety behaviors. As I said then, this is one of the most common things I see that keeps people stuck in the loop. It is crucial that you are aware of the different mental safety behaviors you are engaging in and work to eliminate them.

6. In **Chapter 6**, we explored the concept of consciousness and the importance of understanding your ability to shift into awareness-consciousness. This was probably something you weren't expecting from this book. Still, in my opinion, this is one of the most essential steps in OCD and anxiety recovery, and people (including practitioners!) rarely discuss or include it.

7. In **Chapter 7**, we delved into the Triple-A Response®, including the importance and power of moving into a solution-focused approach instead of focusing on the problem.

8. In **Chapter 8**, we discussed the first step of the Triple-A Response®: "Agree and disengage." As a reminder, here is the central message of this step: **When you agree and disengage the thoughts, you do not agree that what your mind is saying is true. Instead, you simply agree and disengage from whatever your intrusive**

thoughts are saying. You do this to avoid getting caught in the conversation. You do this from a place of awareness-consciousness.

9. In **Chapter 9**, we considered the second step of the Triple-A Response®, "Allow the anxiety." Here is the central message of this step: **When you allow feelings in your body, you are *not* allowing the feeling to make it go away. Instead, you are bringing your awareness into your body and your awareness into the actual feelings and sensations in your body. Then you are giving the feeling permission to come to the surface. Then, when it does, you experience the feeling in its entirety. And just like in step one, you are doing this from a place of awareness-consciousness.**

10. In **Chapter 10**, we chatted about the third step of the Triple-A Response®, "Attacking the anxiety." The central message of this chapter was this: **When attacking anxiety, you move directly toward your intrusive thoughts and anxious feelings. This step's key point is that it comes down to your internal intention. You must attack wholeheartedly. It requires courage and total commitment to move against your resistance to your fear. By doing so, you are dropping all opposition and confronting your fear head-on. And just in steps one and two, you are doing this from a place of awareness-consciousness.**

Let's also review the three main themes of this book:

1. How you understand a problem in life will determine what you do, and what you do will produce specific results. Therefore, if you don't currently have the desired results, you should start by ensuring you understand the problem correctly.

2. The OCD & anxiety loop is not a thought or feeling problem; it is a loop problem, and that loop is fueled by engaging in safety behaviors.

3. Your primary objective for recovery is to break the loop. The best and only way to do that is to eliminate all your safety behaviors, mental and physical. And to do that, you must move to a solution-focused approach called the Triple-A Response®.

Now, at this point, you should have a strong understanding of what you need to do to get started taking your life back from OCD and anxiety. The next step for you is to start putting this into action!

You can decide if you want help or if you want to go it alone. I would highly advise seeking out guidance, as it will condense the amount of time you spend on this journey. But whatever you choose, be sure to start. Make one small decision, and then take one small step.

Your recovery doesn't just happen overnight; it happens because you make the correct behavioral decisions today that ultimately produce a better tomorrow.

The more you decide to do the right things today, the more you will eventually realize that recovery is not some distant place you can't even imagine. Instead, recovery is a choice you make one day at a time. Eventually, if you make the right choice consistently, your recovery will become a present reality you create as a by-product of all the incredible work you put in.

And when that happens, you will only have yourself to thank.

The Triple-A Response® won't remove your intrusive thoughts and anxious feelings, but it will enable you to break the loop, allowing your nervous system to shift into safety, which will allow you to live a more balanced and healthier life. When you live from a state of balance and trust, I believe you can build whatever kind of life you desire.

How I Can Help You

If you *do* want help, there are a few things I can provide. I have broken these down based on where you are on your journey. Just read the statements below and see which one best aligns with you:

"I Am Just Getting Started"

If you are brand new to this and this is the first time you've seen any of my work, I recommend you start by joining **my 2-day intensive workshop: Breaking Free from OCD and Anxiety.**

In this 2-day workshop, I discuss some high-level concepts about OCD and anxiety and go deeper into what you need to start doing to break free from OCD and Anxiety.

On day 1, we cover the following:

- Why everyone commonly misunderstands and mistreats OCD and anxiety issues
- The difference between *solving* and *dissolving* OCD and anxiety
- The complete spectrum of stress and anxiety and how each experience will vary
- All the common mistakes I made (and most people make) that are entirely avoidable
- What it means to be in the "lens" of OCD and anxiety, and, more importantly, how to get out of it

On day 2, we cover the following:

- Why changing your behavior (not your thoughts and feelings) is the key to successfully rewiring your brain
- Why trying to get rid of intrusive thoughts and anxiety is a broken model

- How to uncover limiting beliefs that are keeping you stuck and begin rebuilding new ideas that better serve you
- The importance of moving to a solution-focused process called the Triple-A Response® and why it will help you break out of the loop, reclaim your life, and much more

You can learn more, or join the workshop, by clicking the link below:

https://www.restoredminds.com/breaking-free-workshop

Use the code **SAVE50** at checkout to get $50 off enrollment.

"I Want Clear Guidance and Help Applying the Triple-A Response® and Breaking Out of the Loop"

I recommend joining my Taking Back Control Program if you want step-by-step guidance while working to implement and apply what you learned in this book.

Taking Back Control is my 12-week signature program that takes you from being lost in confusion and chaos to a place of confidence and control by helping you master the Triple-A Response®, so you know exactly what to do mentally, emotionally, and behaviorally without all the guesswork.

Taking Back Control (TBC) was built for anyone struggling with OCD and anxiety, no matter where you are on your journey, combining digital curriculum, coaching, and community. You'll get the clarity, confidence, and support you need to navigate each stage of your recovery.

You can learn more and join Taking Back Control using the link below:
https://www.restoredminds.com/tbc

"I Want to Work with Matt and his Team"

First off, I'm grateful that you are interested in working together. My group and individual coaching programs include LIFETIME access to all of my content and direct access to me and my team. The majority of my coaching programs are conducted online, so my team and I are able to meet with people from all over the world. If you want personalized guidance and coaching while working to implement and apply what you learned in this book, then this option is for you, as this is the highest level of support I can provide you. In addition to coaching, I also offer live private training and workshops.

To learn more and get started, all you need to do is complete our short application form. Then my team and I will review it and reach out to you with the next steps. There's no commitment at all. You've got nothing to lose and everything to gain.

You can complete your application on the link below:
www.restoredminds.com/apply

If you are struggling and want to get your life back, we would be honored to help you however we can.

With that said, I thank you for reading this book, and from the bottom of my heart, I wish you a full recovery and a life not controlled by fear.

To your success,

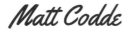

References

American Psychological Association. (2011, October 1). "Suppressing the 'White Bears.'" Monitor on Psychology, 42(9). https://www.apa.org/monitor/2011/10/unwanted-thoughts.

Anxiety and Depression Association of America (n.d.). "Anxiety Disorders—Facts and Statistics." Retrieved 31 October 2022, from https://adaa.org/understanding-anxiety/facts-statistics.

Coelho, P. (1995). *The Alchemist*. Thorsons.

Ekman, P. (1999). "Basic Emotions." In T. Dalgleish and M. J. Power's *Handbook of Cognition and Emotion* (pp. 45-60). Wiley.

Hanson, C. (Director). (2002). *8 Mile* [Film]. Universal Pictures; Imagine Entertainment; RLJE Films.

Hawkins, D. R. (2013). Letting Go: The Pathway of Surrender. Hay House.

Jung, C. G. (2014). Collected Works of C. G. Jung, Volume 8: Structure and Dynamics of the Psyche. Princeton University Press.

Levine, P. A., Frederick, A. (1997). Waking the Tiger: Healing Trauma: The Innate Capacity to Transform Overwhelming Experiences. North Atlantic Books.

Lexico Dictionaries. (n.d.). "Emotion." Retrieved 2 November 2022, from

https://web.archive.org/web/20211009004612/https://www.lexic
o.com/definition/emotion.

Maté, G. (2019). *When the Body Says No: The Cost of Hidden
Stress*. Scribe Publications Pty Limited.

McLeod, S. (2018, October 8). "Pavlov's Dogs." Simply Psychology.
Retrieved 3 November 2022, from
https://www.simplypsychology.org/pavlov.html.

Mental Health Foundation. (n.d.). "Physical Health and Mental
Health." Retrieved 2 November 2022, from
https://www.mentalhealth.org.uk/explore-mental-health/a-z-
topics/physical-health-and-mental-health.

Moorjani, A. (2022). *Dying to Be Me* (10th Anniversary Edition: My
Journey from Cancer, to Near Death, to True Healing.) Hay
House, Incorporated.

Porges, S. W., and Dana, D. (Eds.). (2018). Clinical Applications of
the Polyvagal Theory: The Emergence of Polyvagal-Informed
Therapies. W. W. Norton and Company.

Price, J. R. (2003). *Nothing Is Too Good to Be True*. Hay House.

Robbins, T. [@TonyRobbins]. (2020, May 14). "Where FOCUS goes,
energy flows! Remember, what we FEEL is a result of what we're
choosing to FOCUS on." Twitter.
https://twitter.com/tonyrobbins/status/1260996746672365568?
lang=en-GB.

Roosevelt, F. D. (1933, March 4). *First Inauguration Speech*.
History Matters. http://historymatters.gmu.edu/d/5057/.

Rowling, J. K. (2018). Harry Potter and the Sorcerer's Stone. Bloomsbury.

Sapolsky, R. M. (2004). Why Zebras Don't Get Ulcers: The Acclaimed Guide to Stress, Stress-Related Diseases, and Coping (Third Edition). Henry Holt and Company.

Satpute, A., Wilson-Mendenhall, C., Kleckner, I., and Barrett, L. (2015). "Emotional Experience." *Brain Mapping*, 65–72. https://doi.org/10.1016/b978-0-12-397025-1.00156-1.

Saxena, S., Gorbis, E., O'Neill, J., Baker, S. K., Mandelkern, M. A., Maidment, K. M., Chang, S., Salamon, N., Brody, A. L., Schwartz, J. M., and London, E. D. (2008). "Rapid Effects of Brief Intensive Cognitive-Behavioral Therapy on Brain Glucose Metabolism in Obsessive-Compulsive Disorder." *Molecular Psychiatry, 14*(2), 197–205. https://doi.org/10.1038/sj.mp.4002134.

Schwartz, J. M. and Gladding, R. (2012). You Are Not Your Brain: The 4-Step Solution for Changing Bad Habits, Ending Unhealthy Thinking, and Taking Control of Your Life. Avery.

Siegel, D. J. (2018). Aware: The Science and Practice of Presence—a Complete Guide to the Groundbreaking Wheel of Awareness Meditation Practice: The Science and Practice. Penguin Publishing Group.

Simpson, H., and Hezel, D. (2019). "Exposure and Response Prevention for Obsessive-Compulsive Disorder: A Review and New Directions." *Indian Journal of Psychiatry, 61*(7), 85. https://doi.org/10.4103/psychiatry.indianjpsychiatry_516_18.

Singer, M. A. (2020). The Untethered Soul Lecture Series: Volume 3: The Clarity of Witness Consciousness [CD]. Sounds True.

Van der Kolk, B. A. (2014). The Body Keeps the Score: Brain, Mind, and Body in the Healing of Trauma. Penguin Publishing Group.

van Hout, W. J., and Emmelkamp, P. M. (2002). "Exposure in Vivo Therapy." *Encyclopedia of Psychotherapy*, 761–768. https://doi.org/10.1016/b0-12-343010-0/00091-x.

Weg, A. H. (2011). OCD Treatment Through Storytelling: A Strategy for Successful Therapy. Oxford University Press.

Wegner, D. M. (1994). White Bears and Other Unwanted Thoughts: Suppression, Obsession, and the Psychology of Mental Control. Viking/Penguin.

Wikipedia contributors. (2022, October 26). "Emotion." Wikipedia. https://en.wikipedia.org/wiki/Emotion.

Willink, J. (Host). (2020-present). *Life Is Hard. 12 Rules for Life.* [Audio podcast]. YouTube. https://www.youtube.com/watch?v=WHZjcfgk4Cl.

Won, E., and Kim, Y. K. (2016). "Stress, the Autonomic Nervous System, and the Immune-kynurenine Pathway in the Etiology of Depression." *Current Neuropharmacology, 14*(7), 665–673. https://doi.org/10.2174/1570159x14666151208113006.

Zohuri, B. (2018). "First Law of Thermodynamics." *Physics of Cryogenics*, 119–163. https://doi.org/10.1016/b978-0-12-814519-7.00005-7

Made in United States
Cleveland, OH
22 October 2024

10213911R00090